MW01127955

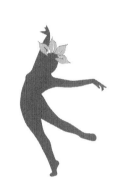

THE DANCING HERBALIST

Wellness for A Moving World

www.thedancingherbalist.com

www.thedancingherbalist.wordpress.com

Facebook: The Dancing Herbalist

Facebook: The Dancing Herbalist's Herbies

Twitter: DanceHerbalist

info@thedancingherbalist.com

A Beginner's Guide to Wellness

The Dancing Herbalist's Wellness Division

Developed for use by clients of The Dancing Herbalist and other wellness practitioners

Jillian Carnrick; MS HM, ACSM CPT

Edited by Kelly 'Kat' Thulen and Xan Hall

Photography by Kirk Zutell and Lia Robinson

Special thanks to: Betsy Miller, Jasper Wolfe, Quinn Wu, Alecks Ferguson, Marilyn Moor, Tanisha Armstrong, Erin Gum, Katie Kraus

For Novella and Norman Rogers.

Thank you for always opening my mind to the natural world around me

And showing me how to love and care for those in it.

-Jillian

CONTENTS

HOW TO USE THIS BOOK

Welcome to the Wellness 101 Workbook. This workbook is designed to walk you through a period of several months to learn more about your own body, and how you can make choices in your daily life to feel better about both your physical and mental wellbeing. Work through this book to find support in hydration techniques, nourishment, movement practices, sleep support, as well as meditation and personal spiritual exploration.

As you begin, you will want to have a designated journal to use for your work through this book. Each chapter includes a variety of small quizzes and critical thinking questions for you to answer to help guide a change in your awareness of your body. You will notice that the questions in this book are all italicized to help highlight them for you to answer in your journal. It is recommended that you do answer these questions, as they will help guide you to learn more about your own body, and in finding what changes will be most effective at supporting your own wellness.

You may want to see the questions and pause to think about them. I recommend taking time to process and write down an answer to each one. When you write things down they become concrete thoughts and beliefs. It is sometimes hard to accept what we are doing to our bodies and minds. This work should be a process of acceptance and acknowledgment of where you are so you are able to see the changes over time. Take the time. Make the commitment to yourself.

You may notice that some of the questions throughout this book are a bit repetitive sounding. This is to help you try to think about the same topic from a different angle. Some of the questions in this book might make you cry or get angry at yourself if it touches on something that is important to you. These are good moments to note in your journal; clear emotional reactions can be very helpful in making the change we want to see in ourselves. Again, take the time with each question, even the repetitive ones, and see what differences they can evoke in you.

Many chapters also have homework assignments in them. You can find a full list of these assignments in appendix D. Most of these will require additional journaling in your book, or you can choose to print a variety of worksheets from **www.thedancingherbalist.com** to support your journaling. You may choose to create a binder to include all of these handouts, so they are in one location. You will not want to lose them as many of the homework assignments will be reviewed in later chapters.

There is a significant amount of science in this book, but you will not be overwhelmed with it. It is included to support your learning your own body. In the back of this book there is a glossary that will help you with words that may be unfamiliar to you. I have tried to be as thorough as possible in including all words that may be unfamiliar but they may not all be there. Personally, I think it is very valuable to know how my own body is working and I recommend that if a word you do not understand is in this book, please look it up. It will support your own personal learning about yourself.

You may notice, as you are completing the work in this book, that many of your larger challenges may not been addressed enough to 'cure' your symptoms. Overcoming many health care challenges cannot be done with wellness practices alone. Many doctors may recommend more exercise for your high blood pressure, but they are going to still put you on drugs to lower it, while you start exercising. This book is intended to set you on the right path to finding what works best for your body. It is highly recommended that as you work through this book you also choose to work with a Certified Nutrition Specialist, Personal Trainer, Herbalist, Naturopathic Doctor, or any other professional in the areas you are in need of additional support. In this book's appendixes, you can find resources to help you find individuals to best support you on your wellness path.

You will notice that the final chapter in this book focuses on herbs to support wellness. I myself am an herbalist with a Master of Science Degree in Herbal Medicine. That does not mean I know everything there is to know about herbs, and I do still recommend you use herbs with caution. There are many potential interactions with pharmaceuticals that herbs can have and none of the herbal recommendations in this book are intended to diagnose or treat any illness. While they can be supportive of your normal wellness practices, herbs are drugs too, and should also be used cautiously and with the direct supervision of a professional herbalist.

If you are interested in learning more about beginner herbal medicine please visit **www.thedancingherbalist.com** where there are a number of free online herbal classes, information about herbal products, and our wellness consultations. We also post twice a week on our blog, **www.thedancingherbalist.wordpress.com** about both herbs and wellness. Not only can you find The Dancing Herbalist on Facebook, but we also have an online discussion group on Facebook called 'The Dancing Herbalist's Herbies.' Please consider following us to continue your own wellness path.

If you are experiencing a medical emergency, are in danger, are feeling suicidal, call 911 immediately.

Suicide Hotline: 800-784-2433
Immediate Medical Assistance: 911
Crisis Call Center: 800-273-8255 or text ANSWER to 839863

CHAPTER 1: WELLNESS INPUTS

We are going to start this off full steam! So, let's talk about what wellness is. What do you think? You have probably heard this word a lot at this point already, so you probably already know something about wellness. In your journal, start to explore the following:

What does wellness mean to you?

What are your 'pillars of wellness'?

Wellness:

The quality or state of being healthy in body and mind, especially as the result of deliberate effort.

An approach to healthcare that emphasizes preventing illness and prolonging life, as opposed to emphasizing treating diseases.

How does this resonate with you?

What are you currently doing to support your own body's wellness? What about your mind wellness?

What are you doing to prevent illness?

Wellness is all about making a conscious choice to serve your body and mind.

Sound's easy, right? I want to make it clear that *wellness is a choice*. A choice to take control of your life, a choice to add sustenance to your life, and a choice to change the quality of your life. You get to choose each time when you eat something, go to bed, or get in your car to do it in a way that is going to help you, or to hurt you. You already make the choice not to eat rocks, right? That is for your wellness. You make sure to sleep with the lights off. This is a choice you make so you can sleep better. Do you get into your car and drive safely? This is a choice we can make to support our own wellness, to keep us well in body and mind.

There are a variety of pillars to wellness that we can think of, pieces that together make up all of the things that keep your body well. I have set up my system with five pieces to make it simple: hydration, nourishment, movement, sleep, and mental wellbeing. I also recommend exploring your environment, the people and places around you, as a sixth pillar to your wellness. You can split your life up in any way you wish that makes it easier for you to separate and care for yourself. This book is meant to be a guide book to get you started in your personal wellness care. Take it a chapter at a time and you will soon, develop your own wellness practices.

I know you can do it! It takes time but we can all make changes in our lives to help create the well person we want to be.

All it takes is that first step.

That first choice to make a difference in our lives, to get us moving. Let's start with food.

FOOD!

Most everyone likes to start with food. And who wouldn't, really? Food is the main thing that affects our wellness.

Why do we eat?

Biologically, we eat because we need food as a fuel source. It is more than that, but let's start there. There are three main groups of chemicals we get from food: carbohydrates, proteins, and fats. Do you know what the following are made of?

Carbohydrates, Proteins, or Fats?

Look at the following and decide if each of them could be described as a carbohydrate, protein, and/or a fat

Ham	Sugar	Bread	Tomato
Cheese	Ice Cream	Black Beans	French Fries
Cucumber	Salsa	Tea/Coffee	Dark Chocolate

Carbohydrates:
Sugar, Bread, Tomato, Cucumber, Ice Cream, Black Beans, French Fries, Salsa, Dark Chocolate, Tea/Coffee

Proteins:
Ham, Cheese, Ice Cream, Black Beans

Fats:
Ham, Cheese, Ice Cream, French Fries

Did they surprise you at all? That easily could be all of the food you eat for a day, right? Most of the things there are carbohydrates and are used by the body all the same way. So what does our body do with carbohydrates? Carbohydrates are the fuel we always are hearing about. Carbohydrates are specifically sugar molecules, and we all know that sugar gives us energy. Not all carbohydrate sugars work the same, but they all give us the energy our cells need to work.

Our bodies primarily use proteins to repair our body. We are made of proteins, and we need the amino acids, building blocks of all proteins, to repair our tissues. This is why proteins are important to eat. You can't heal a broken bone or a cut in your arm without protein. Have you ever wondered why some individuals who are vegan look, well, like death? Many vegans do not choose to get enough protein and then their bodies slowly fall apart. There are healthy, tasty ways to get all of proteins you need from your food. Vegans need to supplement with added amino acids and vitamins for those that do not naturally appear in vegetable plants. There are healthy and non-healthy ways to be a vegetarian or vegan without animal proteins.

Fats are what keep us moving. When you get a massage, you use lotion or oil to make the skin move more easily; this is exactly what happens in the body as well. Fats make up every cell in our body, and make it so we are able to move without getting stuck. Our fats lubricate our joints, as well as our individual tissues, to move against each other. Fats are in the membranes of our cells so that they are able to slide across each other as needed. In the cell walls, fats also help to create a barrier so that things cannot pass through unless they have a transport vehicle. This reduces invaders getting into our cells when they are not meant to. Fats create a barrier to help protect our cells and help our body to move, making them essential to our lives.

Let's start with a few questions to get you thinking about what food means to you.

Why do you eat food?

How does food make you feel physically?

How does food make you feel emotionally?

Do some foods make you tired or energetic?

Are there certain foods you like to have when you are feeling negative?

Are there certain foods you like to have when you are feeling positive?

What is your favorite meal? Why?

Did any of your answers surprise you? Are you happy with your choice of your favorite meal? I am always amazed at how our mood can affect what we eat. What we eat also changes when we are in different moods, but more on that in a bit.

How does food make you feel?

Food can affect both our physical body as well as our emotional wellbeing. Do you know how food makes your body feel? Most people do not. Let's start with a simple practice to check in with how our body feels in response to food.

Sit where you are now and think about how your body is feeling. How are you sitting? Do you have any pains anywhere? Are you a comfortable temperature? Do your clothes feel comfortable? Are you breathing?

Now start to think about what you are going to have for dinner tonight. Will you be having a burger with cheese and lots of ketchup? A salad with crisp lettuce and vine ripe tomatoes? A nice steaming bowl of soup with root vegetables? Dessert? Chocolate, bread pudding, chai or coffee? Walk over to the refrigerator or kitchen, if you are able, and look at the food you have. Smell it and touch it.

Walk away from the food and check in with your body again. Is your mouth watering? Are you feeling pains in your stomach? Are you itching to start to prepare dinner now? Do you have a smile on your face, or are you getting anxious?

Food, and even thinking about food, can directly affect our physiology. Before we even start to eat food we start to experience it and our body gets ready to accept food and digest it. This is why our mouths water when we start to think about food. This preparation is a necessary step of digestion and is just one of the many challenges with eating meals on the go.

Some of you may not start to feel your mouth watering when you think about food. One reason for this may be that your digestion is stalled in a way. Our bodies should be starting the digestive process with just the thought of food, preparing our bodies to receive food. When you do not have this experience, your body may have a harder time breaking down and absorbing the nutrients you need from your food.

The chapters on conscious eating go much deeper into this phenomenon, but for now let's just remember that food can affect both our physical and emotional state. By paying attention to our responses we can make a choice to eat something, or not eat something, based on the physical and emotional reaction we get from the food. This is a great place to just start educating yourself without making any changes to support your wellness.

Just start paying attention to how things make you feel.

HYDRATION INTRODUCTION

Does everyone drink 8 glasses of water a day? YES! Oh, good, we can skip this section. Oh, were you lying? Many people do not get nearly enough water a day. I know that I do not and I work hard to do it too. Our chapter on water will look more closely at a few things you can do to get more water in your life, but let's start with a little about water and why we need it.

Why do we need to drink water?

What does water do in our bodies?

What does it feel like when you have not had enough water?

What does it feel like when you have had too much water?

What is your favorite way to try to get more water?

What is stopping you from having more water on a daily basis?

We all hear that water is important in our bodies, but why? When you drink water, it goes into your stomach where it helps to digest your food. Water is known as the universal solvent. It supports enzymes that break down food in your digestive tract, allowing for more effective nutrient absorption. Water can also be a transport molecule to help bring water soluble vitamins into your body as they are absorbed after digestion.

Once the water has been absorbed by the intestines along with everything else you absorb, it goes to your liver. Water is helpful in your liver to help enzymes to create new proteins and other molecules needed by the body. The water then passes into your circulatory system, your blood, where it directly affects your blood pressure. When someone has high blood pressure they are often given a diuretic to try to remove some of the water from their blood to lower the pressure. When taking a diuretic, you should drink even more water to counteract the extra removal of water from your system. You do not necessarily need to be drinking 8 glasses a day. You may need more, or less. The chapters on hydration will help you observe how your body changes with different amounts of water to find what works best for you. Personally, being an individual with low blood pressure, I need even more water than the average person for my body to be healthy.

Water is the primary solvent in your blood as well. Everything in your blood is floating in a water based fluid. When you do not have enough water your blood can become 'sticky' and will not flow as swiftly. This can reduce your healing capacity, along with reducing other processes that need nutrient delivered to the site of action.

This only happens with severe dehydration, but it is important to note that this stickiness also appears in our mucus, and is one reason we are told to drink fluids when we are sick. With more liquids, our mucus will remain more fluid and help to flush out more disease particles from our nose. This goes for other mucous membranes as well, but the others are generally more difficult to see.

When water gets to our cells it is transported inside and helps to create a fluid environment wrapped in the fats you have eaten. Again, most of the molecules inside of our cells work with the assistance of water for enzymes and transportation mechanisms. Water can also be used to help draw waste out of a cell, and into the space between cells in our bodies. These wastes and the water, are picked back up by the circulatory system to be flushed out of the body. Our kidneys use an osmotic balance set up against water, to pull waste compounds out of our blood along with some water, to dilute our urine.

The more water that is in your blood the more toxins you are able to pull out with your kidneys for urination. Similarly, you can see in your urine if you are drinking enough water to support this process. If your urine is clear to pale yellow, you are good. Having a darker yellow urine on a regular basis can be a sign of a potential infection or simply a sign that you need to be drinking more water. Be sure to pay attention and see a doctor if you are concerned.

Other signs that you should be drinking more water is if your mouth is dry, if you get headaches, or are dizzy frequently. Your mouth being dry is not only a sign that you should drink water in that moment, it is a sign that you are generally not getting enough water. It takes a little time to set up a water balance so that your mucus membranes are fluid with enough water, so when you are thirsty, it is too late to shift the balance for that moment. Similarly, if you spray when you talk, or if you can see saliva in your mouth when you talk you need more water.

MOVEMENT INTRODUCTION

Now, again, most of us do not get enough movement in our lives either. But that is alright. We all have busy lives and through this book we will continue to give you tools to help you find ways to add these wellness inputs into your life more effectively. Movement is one of those things that people often just do not like. It is work in itself, so I do not blame you for wanting to just skip this section right now. I would highly advise against this. Let's just start with a little true and false quiz.

True   False

_____ _____ Sitting in the office all day does not have any positive or negative effects. It is neutral.

_____ _____ Walking is a great way to start exercising.

_____ _____ Walking is an excellent way to get all of the exercise you need.

_____ _____ Movement does **not** help with detoxing our body.

_____ _____ Moving is not good for heart wellness.

_____ _____ Running is necessary for circulatory support from movement.

_____ _____ Wiggling is a valid form of movement.

_____ _____ If you exercise properly, you will not get injured.

_____ _____ Exercise causes stress and anxiety.

_____ _____ Exercising hurts.

_____ _____ Exercising can be fun and enjoyable.

Answers:

FALSE Sitting in the office all day does not have any positive or negative effects. It is neutral.

Sitting itself can be detrimental to your health. It is being suggested that sitting for 2-3 hours in a row will negate the beneficial effects of 30 minutes of vigorous movement. This suggests that just standing to do your everyday tasks such as computer work will be better for you than sitting.

TRUE Walking is a great way to start exercising.

Yes, it sure is. If you are used to sitting all day and you need to start moving in some way, then walking is a great way to get onto your feet. Don't forget, when you see this little walking person throughout this book, take a few minute break to get up and walk around. This is an easy way to add in a few more minutes of movement each day.

FALSE Walking is an excellent way to get all of the exercise you need.

Unfortunately, walking does not meet the standards of movement suggested by the American College of Sports Medicine. It is suggested that three 30-minute exercise bouts a week, of moderate to vigorous activity is a minimum place to be at for movement wellness. Ideally, they suggest that you do five 30 minute bouts a week. We will get there. Just start with walking until you are ready for more.

FALSE Movement does not help with detoxing our body.

Movement is a great way to help your body detoxify. It works for this through two different methods. First of all, we know that when we are doing moderate to vigorous activity, we start to sweat. Sweating is one of the ways that our body releases toxins through our skin.

The other way typical movement helps to detoxify your body is by helping to move your lymph fluid through your body. Your lymphatic system collects a variety of toxic substances and flushes them out of your body through your digestive tract. The challenge with the lymph system is that there is no muscle tissue to move the toxins to the digestive tract. Rather the lymphatic system uses all your movement to push the toxins through your body.

FALSE Moving is not good for heart wellness.

Most exercise focuses on working the muscles and yes, the heart is a muscle. Slowly increasing movement and exercise helps to increase the strength and endurance of the heart muscle itself. This comes by simply practicing using the heart muscle at a higher capacity, through moderate exercise.

FALSE Running is necessary for circulatory support from movement.

Vigorous movement is not necessary for circulatory support. Moderate energy movement is all that is needed, but over time you can build a tolerance to this. You may need to increase your energy expenditure to get the same results. There are also plenty of other ways to exercise other than running to get the energy expenditure needed for the benefits to your circulatory system. Other moderate to vigorous activities that are great include swimming, dancing, biking, and a variety of strengthening exercises.

TRUE Wiggling is a valid form of movement.

Wiggling is an excellent way to move. It is ideal to support lymphatic flow and it can be fun! Often wiggling or creative self-dancing is one of the best ways to start moving. Doing it alone in your home is a great way to build your own confidence around movement. I love to wiggle. Though it sounds funny, you know it would be fun to do too.

FALSE If you exercise properly you will not get injured.

Even the best athletes get injured sometimes. The more you get used to moving, and the stronger and more flexible you become, the more you reduce your risk of getting injured doing everyday things. For instance, if you reach too high and hurt your shoulder, it could have been prevented if you had been stretching regularly and were used to moving your shoulder in that fashion. Similarly, hurting your back by picking up a heavy box, could be prevented if you had already strengthened your back muscles through movement.

FALSE Exercise causes stress and anxiety.

It is true that for some people, thinking about exercise can be stressful. Doing the actual exercise may feel stressful at first, in the long term will actually reduce your stress experience. Exercise releases endorphins to reduce your stress response rather than causing it.

The more you exercise the more you enjoy it.

TRUE Exercising hurts.

There are three different ways that exercise can hurt. The most obvious is if you get injured. Second, if you are not used to doing an exercise, whether it be strengthening or stretching, doing the actual exercise can be painful. With this pain, the more you do it the easier it will become and over time, less painful.

The third pain comes after exercising. This is called delayed onset muscle soreness (DOMS) which shows up 24-48 hours after exercising. DOMS occurs when your body is inflamed after exercise and the tissues then get damaged from the inflammation, causing the pain. A way to prevent this, once you are doing consistent exercise, and are experiencing this phenomenon, is to focus on reducing your body's inflammatory response to exercise by following some of the tips in the chapter on inflammation.

TRUE Exercising can be fun and enjoyable.

Exercising, of course, can be enjoyable. No one says you have to do exercise that you do not find fun. Find a friend to exercise with. Enjoy the outdoors while exercising. Listen to music or read a book while at the gym on a treadmill. If you don't want to go to a gym there are great ways to exercise at home, too. Videos on YouTube can help you find new movements. Try laughing yoga for instance and laugh your way to starting more movement. Crank up the music and start to enjoy your movement!

SLEEP INTRODUCTION

Do I need to ask? No, few of us get enough sleep. We already know that. Everyone always says get 7-10, or about 8 hours, of sleep a night, but we never find the time to do that. Why do we need sleep in the first place?

Why do YOU sleep?

What happens to your body when you sleep?

How do you feel when you wake up?

What would a healthy sleep schedule for YOU be?

What would be the benefit for you to have a consistent sleep schedule?

What is stopping you from having the sleep schedule you want?

Sleep is something we all need. There are stories of a variety of famous people not sleeping for more than 20 minutes a day. Only one in a million people can do this, and for the rest of us, we need more sleep. Sleep is our primary method or recharging our batteries. We use the time sleeping to digest food, build new tissues, repair injuries, and detoxify our bodies.

The other big thing we do while sleeping is dream. We use our dreams to process the events of the day, and they are essential to digesting the stresses we deal with. Dreams allow our bodies to enact situations we may need to mentally process and explore more, often giving us insight to our own reasons for our actions. While not everyone needs or benefits from this mental processing, it is a key reason that having adequate sleep benefits our stress levels.

Sleep is also necessary to recharge our mental capacities. When you are not getting enough sleep, you are damaging your nervous tissue and preventing it from repairing itself while you sleep. Caffeine can be a temporary fix to this, but long term it can be very detrimental to your mental and physical health, with your body not having the time to heal and strengthen your nervous tissue during sleep.

Your mental capacity includes your reaction time as well. This is especially important when driving. Driving while being tired can be just as bad as driving while intoxicated. Do not be afraid to pull over if you are tired. I have done this, and I have had a variety of experiences with it. Once, I had a police officer come and wake me up and tell me to get off of the highway if I was going to sleep in my car. This is one dilemma you may face, but there is always a safe place, and if an officer is upset for where you are sleeping they should be able to offer you another option.

When trying to get the sleep you need there are a few basic strategies you can take. The first thing that I tried was scheduling when I was going to go to sleep along with other daily activities. It was challenging, but by having a more detailed sleep schedule, when I was going to get things done, having a space for extra activities, and a set time to stop doing each activity, I was a little more able to stop what I was doing and prepare for bed. Also, having a ritual before going to bed of brushing your teeth, turning lights down an hour before bed, and reading a book are all good steps to take to prepare for sleeping.

PERSONAL ENVIRONMENT

This pillar of wellness regards your home, work, the people around you in these places, your outdoor experiences, and other communities you are involved with. The main reason that I am including these in our main pillars of wellness is that they are the most common stress as causing things in our lives: work, relatives, and home life. Most of us know the primary events that cause us stress. What can we do with our environment to reduce our stress?

Are there individuals you are frequently around that effect your wellness? How?

Are there places that you do not feel quite yourself? Why?

Home

Have a place separate from everything else that is your space. Even if that is just a chair or an office desk, or a whole separate room, have a space where you can separate yourself from the people looking for your attention or from the things that need to be done. Having an activity to do at home to take a break is also a good idea. Possibilities here include having a book to read, taking a bath, meditating, having a place to do some exercise, or taking a break to watch a television show. Some people need a quiet home to relax and having a separate quiet space can be helpful. Others need noise, and having the television or radio on can be supportive. What helps to relieve your stress and how can you add that into your home life?

Work

We all work in different environments and we all work 'well' in different environments. Create an environment in your work space that is conducive to how you work best. Taking breaks is important and the law requires that you do so. If your employer does not offer them to you, ask! It is important to your own wellness. It can also be difficult to work with some people. Not everyone has the same views of how the work place should be run. The best way to deal with your upsets regarding this is to talk to your supervisor about how you should handle challenges. When they appear to be personal problems, calmly talking to the other people involved can sometimes solve the challenge.

Though it sounds silly to most adults, really putting yourself into their shoes can make a big difference in how you interpret and react to a situation. Similarly, meditation and relaxation techniques can really reduce your stress response when someone pushes your buttons. There are more tools to help with this in our chapter on stress.

Relatives and Partners

Ah, the joy of others! A cause of stress for everyone at some level. Your family are the people that know you best, and often provide some of the most challenging relationships through our lives. They are there through your ups and downs, and boy can that be stressful, as you are there for theirs as well. Taking the time to check in with the people around you to see what they need is a great tool to show them that you care and to help reduce their stress.

It can also help to know that you are supporting their needs, reducing their upsets, often the source of your stress. When they are not stressed or worried, they will be less likely to take their upset out on others. This opens up space for your own wellbeing. When you have relatives visiting your home, it is all right to designate a space where they cannot go, in some fashion. This will give you a way to separate yourself from them if needed.

There are also environments that can be stress reducing for us as well. These should be used as tools for when we need a little relaxation or a break from stressful environments. Ideally we would be trying to shift our home and work lives so that they do not have stress causing agents, and that they are full of communication and openness. These sorts of environments are great to bring a piece of peace into your home or work place.

Community

Having a social community outside of your family is a great stress reliever to most people, and it can be a great place to develop other areas of your life that can feel like they are restricted at home or work. Often we look to our community outside of our home as a place to escape, a place to go to for pleasure and to be around others with similar interest as ours. This can be very fulfilling, but should be something to strive for in our home and work lives as well, a place where we can be fully ourselves and still participate in the event at hand.

Nature and the Outdoors

Now, nature and the outdoors is not a good place for everyone, but if it is one for you, you should get out and enjoy it. Spending time outside in a forest can be beneficial to one's health. This is because of the cleaner air and light spectrum we experience there. Some people find their spiritual inspiration when they are in nature, and are invigorated there as a result. Where do you feel spiritually invigorated and inspired? Use this as a tool to support your wellness.

What are the positives and negatives to each environment you find yourself in?

What can be changed to support you in each environment?

What struggles do you experience with others?

What steps can you take now to improve these relationships?

MAKING A SCHEDULE

One of the biggest things that has helped me in my work and home life to reduce stress has been making a schedule. It takes a lot of effort each week to plan when you are going to do everything, but it is also a way to set your priorities straight and to really schedule in all of the things you want to do to support your own wellness. I always use Google Calendar but there are many other ways you can keep a schedule. I like that application because I can have it on my phone, it is attached to my e-mail, I can share calendars with other people, and I can have events repeat every week with a simple click.

I make sure to schedule in when I am going to be working, eating, sleeping, driving, exercising, socializing, as well as all of my other small chores that I need to do. I also schedule in a time to do next week's schedule. This tool was great in getting me started in moving towards wellness. I may not complete all of my wellness tasks each week but I know that they have a place in my schedule. When I am ready to make the change on an individual task, I do not need to find a time or the tools to make it happen.

Accepting that I might not get to all of my wellness practices every week has been very relaxing for me. This ability to be flexible with my schedule has served me in developing my schedule into more of a routine. A routine to your day is something you do without much thought. Having my wellness practices scheduled into my life has encouraged them to become part of my everyday life, making the commitment to them easier.

We have gone through a wide variety of different health and wellness inputs here and barely scratched the surface of how you can use each one to support your individual wellness needs. Please continue to support your own wellness path by continuing with this book. Even if you only have gotten one thing out of these pages so far you are already started on a new path to better yourself for a longer, happier, more well lifestyle.

INSPIRATIONAL ACTIVITIES

Now we are going to backtrack a little bit. I think one of the key pieces to everyone's wellness is feeling inspired. For many people this comes through spiritual practices. For others it comes through a successful business, or through friends and family. I feel that it is important to have these connections to keep us going and to get to the places we want to be in in life. It is hard to move forward if you are not thankful and accepting of the place you are in now. Let's take a look at where you are in life and where you want to be.

What pieces of your life make you happy?

What pieces of your life do not make you happy?

What is your ideal method of making a living for yourself?

What is your favorite hobby?

What are you proud of that you have done?

What are your personal beliefs about life?

What do you need in your life to be happy?

Do you have these things? Can you add them?

Where do you feel most yourself?

What do you like most about yourself?

What is your passion in life?

What steps are you currently taking towards your life's passion?

What are your goals for the next year?

What are your goals for the next five years?

What will make you most happy if you add it to your life tomorrow?

This is a self-explorative process. Feel free to go back over these questions regularly to see what has changed about your life outside of your physical wellness needs. We so often disregard our mental wellness and it is really the puzzle piece that allows us to go through our day without hurting ourselves or others through our words and actions. Having good mental health can not only serve you well, but also serve your entire community when you offer clear communication without judgements.

CHAPTER 2: BEHAVIOR CHANGE AND MEETING YOUR GOALS

At this point, I am sure you have already begun to look at your wellness in a different light. Now the real challenge is how to add them to your life as you begin to learn more about your own body and wellness capabilities. When we add new behaviors to our lives there are five main steps we take along the way. Do not get discouraged if you feel challenged in one of the steps. It is very common to go back and forth between the first three stages until you are ready to jump to the fourth stage. When you are ready, you will move on to the next step. The main activity that I see that helps people work towards their wellness aspirations is having clear, obtainable goals. We will start with that.

GOALS

If you are ready to make changes, start here and see what kinds of goals you are ready for, and what path to take them along. You may not yet be ready for this, but see what you can do. Then move on to the next section to break it down further to help you find the correct goals for yourself.

What are three goals you have to support your wellness?

Choose one of these goals to start with. Visualize the path you will take to obtain this goal. What are five steps you must take along this path?

Which of these steps are you on right now? What are three things you can do to support yourself on this step?

What can you do TODAY to accomplish one of these steps?

If you had no trouble at all with laying out your goals and knowing how you were going to get there, that is great! That means you are already to move onto the third step of changing a behavior! If you did have some trouble, that's ok, we will now slow down a bit to talk about what behavior change looks like before we have our goals set in place. You will have many opportunities throughout this book to set new goals.

Try not to be overwhelmed with multiple goals and take them one step at a time.

1. PRE-CONTEMPLATION

If you have yet to think about your behavior change, this is the stage you arrive in. In pre-contemplation you are generally starting to learn about the possibilities of things you could change for healthier behavior. This is when you begin to form new social connections so you have the tools to support you when you are ready to make a change. A sign of this is generally when we are looking at new aisles in the grocery store, glancing at bulletin boards we come across, bringing up new ideas to our friends to see if they agree. This is often a time when you will search out new friends and communities that are more in line with the new health values you are starting to understand. At this stage you have not done any of the actual changes to your behavior to support the health change. Think of this as pre-planning.

One of the best tools we can use in this stage of behavior change is making lists of things that you could do to better yourself and the associated positive benefits you can get from each of these things. Use this time to make your list. Stay away from thoughts of where you have been and phrase your benefits in positives of where you are going.

What are ten things you would like to change about yourself?

What positive benefits would you obtain from each of these changes?

Why *do you want to make these behavioral changes?*

Example: I would like to read more.

- Learn more
- Relax
- Engage my brain

I feel better about myself when I read more frequently.

Now, if you actually had ten things you could do to make yourself better, don't consider it to be a lot of work, because we are making a new lifestyle. This is not like going on a diet where you do something for a certain amount of time. Each of these items could easily take a year to implement and fully incorporate into your life. This is not something we can do in a day or even a week. What we are trying to do here is create a new lifestyle where you will constantly be experimenting and trying new things to work towards your constant goal of a healthy and happy lifestyle.

2. CONTEMPLATION

In this stage you are considering what you can do to accomplish the changes you wish to actualize. Generally, you have not yet begun to actually do anything but you are rather starting to think about your goals and how you are going to get there. Let's pick one of the goals you would like to achieve and use that for this stage, and as a guide for the rest of this chapter. Chose something you would actively like to include in your life right now.

What is one goal you can work on throughout this chapter in order to better yourself?

The best goals are developed following the SMART principal. Be **Specific** about your goal. Not just, "I want to get healthy." "I want to be able to lift up my children for ten seconds," is a good one. You want it to be **Measurable**. Losing weight is very general. Losing 10 pounds is a measurable goal and you will know when you have completed that goal. I will also keep talking about making sure your goals are **Attainable**. Having a goal of 4% body fat is just not practical for anyone. You should not drink water and fast for a week. These are extremes. Make sure you can actually accomplish your goal. Your goal also needs to be **Relevant** to your lifestyle. If you work at a grocery store stacking shelves you may not need the extra exercise or strength training, but you may need to work on finding healthy food choices as you have a higher number of food choices available to you and tempting you daily.

Having a **Time Bound** goal is also super important. This is the part that people often get stuck on. Give yourself an amount of time you need to finish each step of your goal. While this is a good method to encourage us to finish, it may discourage us if we cannot do it. I recommend doubling the period of time you have set to meet your goal. If you are unable to complete it in this time pick a new goal. You may not be ready for the first one right now. Try a different aim, review your challenges and come up with new solutions. This is a time to review and update your plan if you are struggling. Having this time frame structure will keep you moving towards your goals when you are stuck.

> SMART Goal Example:
> I will read a leisure book for 30 minutes twice a week,
> for four weeks in a row within a 3-month period.

What is your goal? Be clear in your intentions and make it a SMART goal.

Visualize a path you will take to obtain this goal. What are five steps you must take along this path?

Which of these steps are you on right now? What are three things you can do to support yourself on this step?

What are three things you can do to help you on each of the other steps towards your goal. If you need to break it down further feel free to do so.

> Example: Five Steps to take
>
> 1. Choose a Book
> 2. Find time to read
> 3. Read
> 4. Find another time to read
> 5. Find a consistent time of day to read
>
> Step 4: Three things for support
> 1. Prioritize my schedule
> 2. Commit to finishing other activities
> 3. Remember the rewards to reading

During contemplation we often start to see in our daily lives the consequences of our current behavior. This helps us build a stronger connection to our goals, wanting to get above and beyond the negative side of our behavior. For many of our health-related behaviors we learn about the negative side through wellness and health care facilities. While there are many free online resources that can offer information about your behaviors, you will build a stronger connection with wanting to remove or add a behavior by looking at how you experience the behavior in your own body.

What are five negative results of your current behavior, or lack of a behavior, that you experience?

What are five things stopping you from making the change?

Now look at each of the things stopping you. What can you do with each one of these so it is no longer a reason that stops you from making a change? For instance, if drinking more water is your goal and you don't have any cups, you need to go buy some cups or a water bottle.

Something else that is commonly done in the contemplation stage is visualizing yourself with the changed behavior. This is an excellent way to make an emotional connection to the change. When you are emotionally motivated to make a change it can become much easier to make the change.

How do you view your life being different with this behavior change?

What new possibilities show up in your life with this change? What other goals seem more possible?

3. PREPARATION

Now that you have moved through determining your goals and feel connected to your need for a behavior change you are in the preparation stage. You are 'prepared to change.' This does not mean that you are done and you can just include the behavior consistently now. This means you are ready to start adding changes into your life. Generally, the preparation stage takes about a month of starting and stopping with the plan you have created to meet your goals. If you come across a challenge break it down and find what you can do to overcome that challenge.

When you are finally ready to 'make the change' for good, determine when you are going to do it. Always be able to word your decisions in a positive motivating light to keep you going. Don't say, 'I will just have one last cigarette tonight." Say, "Tomorrow morning I will start being a non-smoker."

When are you going to start your first step?

We have spent a lot of time in this chapter making goals. There is a reason for this. Having clear, easily obtainable goals will help make your path easier to travel and having a large goal you are working towards will inspire you to keep working on all of the steps you have laid out to get there.

Are your goals attainable in a reasonable amount of time? If not, go back and make the changes you need so you can easily accomplish your goals with a little effort.

Often the preparation stage is the time that we have to get rid of old things that are no longer serving us in our new behavior. Getting rid of those cigarettes, tossing the candy you have hiding, clearing a space in your room to exercise. This is the time to be doing all of your preparations. Know how to get in touch with support groups and help hotlines as you might need them.

Have a friend willing to commit to supporting you if you would like the extra encouragement. Make sure they know when you are going to make a change and what you need them to do to support you. Have them check in on you ever few days to see how you are doing. Ask that they make a commitment to checking in. This is an excellent opportunity to also offer to support them with any changes they are struggling through. Having a buddy is always helpful, and helping another also making a change can encourage you to keep working at it as well.

For some individuals, having clear intentions and visualization of separation to a behavior can be very effective at creating a space where new behaviors are able to be accomplished. One of the easiest ways to do this is to take out the trash. As you take out your garbage bag, think about taking your health negative actions and throwing them out with the trash. Sometimes this step involves physical items holding you back. Throw them in the dumpster, watch them get taken away by the truck, see your behaviors leave you of your own free will. You don't need those behaviors anymore; they no longer serve you.

If you are adding new behaviors to your life, visualizing taking in your new behavior, much like eating it, especially if it is related to food. Drink water with the intention of creating a new healthy body within yourself. Think to yourself, "as I drink this water I am improving my life." These self-affirming thoughts when doing your new behavior can be a great motivator as well. If you are thinking "Ugh, I've got to exercise again," you will get nowhere. If you are thinking, "With this push up I will be stronger to pick up my kids," you will get more benefits out of your exercise and new behavior.

What small steps are you going to take over the next two weeks to meet your goals? Write out a daily plan in your journal that you can stick to. Make certain goals and try to keep to them. Don't make them unattainable though. If your goal is to walk three days a week, schedule that in your calendar. Or start with two a week and see if you can do that for two weeks in a row. Start small with things you *can* do. You will feel that your goals are much more attainable if you start slow and work on consistency before trying to go all out and try to jog every day of the week.

Take the time now to outline small steps you can take over the next two weeks towards your larger goal. Consider making a small step every day so you are being both consistent and making movement towards your larger goal.

Look at your plan. Are your goals all SMART goals? If not, go back and clarify them even more.

4. ACTION

As soon as you take that first step out the door to walk, or pick up your fork to eat your first dairy free meal, or pour your first glass of water, you are in the action stage! Congratulations! You have taken the first active step towards your own personal wellness goals. This is a huge step. Be sure to reward yourself somehow.

I love to reward myself with other wellness related activities that may be future goals of mine. If I remembered to drink all of the water I needed for a day I will reward myself with fruit or a relaxing walk outside. This rewards system is self-proliferating and just keeps growing as you reward yourself more. This is not for everyone, and for some a nice bath or an extra ½ hour of television is a great reward. There is nothing that says you cannot do this. I would highly recommend not doing things that could be detrimental to your other areas of wellness, such as rewards with candy or staying up later. Especially for kids, but also adults, this kind of reward system does not set up a full wellness centered lifestyle.

Now that you are in the action stage, don't get too excited. You will probably fall back to one of the first three stages a few times before you move past the action stage. This stage takes minimally six months to move through. That may seem like a long time, but when you think that you only have to focus on one wellness goal through that six-month period, take a sigh of relief. Don't try to do too much at the same time. You do not want to overwhelm yourself. Let one tool become your priority and focus until it becomes second nature and you no longer have to work or remind yourself to do it.

In the action stage commonly you will start to see the benefits of the action you took. Remember the benefits you wanted in the first place? When you start to see these it makes the behavior change even easier on yourself. When this happens we usually start talking about it to our friends. "Did you hear? My blood pressure went down this week and I lost five pounds this month." This is great because, generally, your friends will start to encourage you to keep working at it, seeing how happy you are with your achievement. Keep them around, these friends, and keep building a support system that encourages you to make the change.

What are five benefits you will receive as result of your new behavior?

If your support system is still small, make a public commitment to your new behavior. If you have Facebook or other social media platforms you can post it there. Tell people to hold you to your commitment. If you feel uncomfortable asking people to hold you to your commitment, you may not be ready to make the commitment yet. Having a social network for support is important. When you say out loud, to the world, what you want, you are more likely to make sure it happens.

I, _____, am going to

_____

_____

starting today!

When you make commitments in the action stage, remember that a powerful tool is to set a time limit on it. While this may not sound like it makes sense, having accomplished one day, or even one hour of following your new behavior can be rewarding. If you have a thing you are trying to change, ask yourself these questions:

Could you do it?

Would you do it?

When?

Your answers should be "Yes, Yes, Now!", but if they are not, ask yourself some additional questions when you get stuck in the action phase.

- Could you do it for one week? One day? One hour? Five minutes?
- Would you do it for your family? Would you do it for your kids? Would you do it to help your community? Would you do it to for yourself? Who would benefit from this change?
- Tomorrow? No. In an hour? No. NOW!

Work your way to answer the questions as "Yes, Yes, Now!", making adjustments to your commitment as you go to make this 'NOW' possible. This ability to adjust your commitment for obtainable tasks is what makes this tool good at creating possibilities. Re-making your commitment on a daily basis will help you to achieve the behavior change you wish.

While in the action phase, you may fail many times. This just means you should go back and see if there is a way to prevent each failure from happening again. Write it down, so if it comes up again, you can look back and see what you can do to prevent it from happening. While this is not a surefire way to prevent failure, it can help in some situations.

You can also take the action stage as a time to continue to make your environment more conducive to your new behavior. You may have started this in the preparation stage, but you will find as you go that there are things that will tempt you to slip back into your old habits. For example, I found my worst habit was working on my computer in front of the television. It was harming my posture, I wasn't getting as much exercise, and I was not getting my work done. The change I had to make in my environment was making sure the power cord to my computer was in another room. This change gave me the ability to work in front of the television sometimes, but I would always have to return to my desk, sit with good posture, get up and move around during the day, just so my computer would be at the power cord to charge. Over time, I have found that my posture has improved to a place I am happy with, and I am finding it easier to turn off my television and get the work done that I need to.

The action stage is also a great time to start keeping a journal. Much of this book will include journaling, and I must admit I am still a beginner at journaling my experiences too. I keep practicing and there are times I find journaling extremely helpful, especially when I am trying to observe my relationship with behaviors and experiences. I cannot always remember what I ate at the time, and how I felt in response to it, or how I felt when I did not exercise. Even one or two sentences a day can help jog your memory of what happened on a day, and how you could alter your behaviors to continue to improve your quality of life.

Tracking not only your physical experiences but also your emotional reactions to events can be important. If you notice you are not feeling emotionally stable on days where you accomplish your behavior change, you may not want to keep up with this change even if it just a coincidence. Always make changes as you need, and remember you are in control and have the choice to make if you are going to commit to a new behavior.

5. MAINTENANCE

At this stage you have now been successfully integrating your new behavior change for six months now! In the action stage you get on and off of your behavior change, but once you are on and have been actively participating in your new change for six months, you are now moving into the maintenance phase of your change. You can still fall off the boat, but it will be easier for you to jump back on. By now you are easily seeing the benefits of your behavior change, and this is what is keeping you on the boat.

You may jump on and off of that boat for years now that you have initiated this complete path to behavior change. Remember that it is your choice, and you have the power to affect your own lifestyle and wellness. You have the tools here to go back and forth between each step but always keep looking forward to the person you want to be in your life. You can get there if you really want it, and are prepared to make necessary changes.

COMMON CHALLENGES

Adding New Behaviors

Generally, when we think of behavior change we tend to think about removing behaviors. We think of removing unhealthy food, stopping smoking or drinking alcohol, and similar things. With a wellness model, it is generally easier to make a transition to wellness through adding healthy behaviors rather than thinking of removing unhealthy behaviors. Getting rid of behaviors you enjoy, even if they are health negative, can be difficult for anyone. It is often easier to add new behaviors to your life with the support of the less beneficial habits you already have.

It is easier to add more vegetables to your food intake when you can still eat cake in the evenings. It is easier to get up and get walking if you can still allow yourself a cigarette as a reward. There will be a balance you have to make as you start to incorporate healthy behaviors into your life. You may notice that, over time, you feel better walking when you do not have cigarettes, as walking becomes more important to you. The same goes for that cake. With paying more attention to your food, you may notice that the vegetables make you feel lighter and more energized when sometimes the cake makes you feel tired and sluggish. That does not mean you have to completely take cake out. You have a choice. You can have cake when you want to. You just are aware now of how you will feel in response.

Time

Finding the time to add in new behaviors is often the hardest of all challenges. How do you schedule your life so that you cook a meal at home, get 30 minutes of exercise a day, get 8 hours of sleep, drink a half a gallon of water, and have time for work and your spiritual activities? This is hard! Again, it is choosing what you get the most benefit out of for your current situation. If you work long days and can't get 8 full hours of sleep every night, but if you can eat a healthy diet, you may be able to feel more well than you would if you did not eat nutritiously. On the other hand, you may find that your body needs the extra sleep, and you may take that time away from your food preparation, eating less home cooked foods. Finding the balance you need is the hardest problem. This is why observing how your body reacts to different situations will be an important step as you go through each chapter.

If you do not already have a detailed calendar I recommend making one. For example, I use Google Calendar because I can easily share it with others, color code it, and move dates and times around easily without the scratch marks of pen on paper. Another benefit of Google Calendar is that on each event you can include information such as the location and any other notes you need, things to bring, websites, and contact information. It can also send alarms to your computer, phone, or any other wireless device.

While this may not be the solution for you, I have found that scheduling in time for making food, time for sleeping, exercising, socializing and my work is the only way I can get everything done. I also make sure to schedule in time to relax and to do fun things so I don't get too bogged down or worried about my work. Every Sunday afternoon I have a 3-hour block that all I do is arts and crafts. This is my largest stress reduction tool, so it needs to be part of my schedule in a prominent manner.

One fun way to make a schedule is to start with some graph paper. Decide how many blocks each ½ hour or hour will be. Cut out strips for how long you want or need to do each of your activities: 8 hours for work, 8 hours for sleep, 1 hour for exercise, 2-3 hours daily for cooking and cleaning, 1 hour daily for fun, 1 hour for showering and body care, 1 hour for reading. The fun part is then moving around and trying out the different orders and times for when you are not at work or sleeping. Always start with the big ones and then edit around them. You can also choose to do this over a week-long period if you are not doing every wellness practice every day. Not everyone's needs are going to be the same. Through this book you may need to make changes to your schedule as you learn what works best for you.

Cost

Cost can also be a big inhibitor of adding new behaviors. Most of the behaviors in this book can be altered without too much cost. Sleep, hydration, and exercise can all easily be done without any additional costs. Sometimes with sleep, it may cost us money if we are using over the counter products to help us sleep. With hydration, it can cost us money if we are using fruits or other water additives for our water. Even water filters can be a drain on finances. Some people are dedicated gym goers and only will exercise there. While there are many benefits of working with a personal trainer, it costs money and can easily be something you can remove from your monthly costs. It is possible to help yourself in all of these areas of your wellness without incurring any additional costs.

For some, adding more time for sleep will mean they cannot work as long, and thus reduce their income. Many challenges like this will appear as you work on your wellness. Finding a balance that works for you is important. In this case, it may be that you drop that extra cup of coffee for a week and your sleep quality improves. With this, no extra sleep is needed for the balance to be effective. There is then also one less cup of coffee to purchase. This is a problem-solving game. Weigh your costs and benefits as they specifically pertain to you.

Food really is the one input that directly is affected by the amount of money we can put into it. While I would love everyone to eat organic food it may not be what works best for you right now. If you price compare when you shop, sometimes there are some foods that are less expensive when organic. One common one of these is carrots. When you shop around, there are often places where organic carrots, in large quantities, are cheaper than conventionally grown carrots.

Buying organic does not need to be your first step. What good is buying organic carrots if you don't eat them? Generally, grains are the least expensive, followed by vegetables, with meat as the most expensive. While this is a great reason to become vegetarian, that lifestyle does not work for everyone. Knowing that you can balance monetary costs with the different kinds of food you purchase is important. Also, generally, purchasing whole foods, the actual plants and animals rather than pre-prepared foods, is less expensive.

If you are stuck in the fast food circle due to cost, it is hard to get out. One of the largest motivators to reduce fast food intake is the medical bills. While it is up to you to do your own research and experimenting with your own body, generally people who consume fast food regularly also suffer from diabetes, high blood pressure, low energy, and are significantly overweight. All of these conditions lead to additional costs outside of food preparation. Long term, spending a little more on your food and having better quality whole foods leads to a general reduction in the incidence of these related health challenges.

CHAPTER 3: WATER IN OUR BODIES

Homework Assignment 1

Observe and record the following for a week.

- When do you drink water?
- How much water you drink?
- When do you urinate?
- The color of your urine on a 1-5 scale

Do you notice any patterns?

Did you notice any other symptoms through the week that could be associated with your hydration level?

WHAT IS WATER?

This seems like a very easy question to answer. For some of us it is something we drink, for others it is dihydrogen monoxide, for some it is a river or lake, or a place to swim, exercise in or for a shower. There are also some who see water as a life force, the blood of the earth, and the blood of our body. How can such a small molecule that we usually disregard in our daily lives do so much?

How does water show up in your life?

Have you noticed anything about how your body feels with more or less water?

Is water important to focus on in your life? Why or why not?

PROPERTIES OF WATER

Water is a molecule made with two hydrogen atoms and one oxygen atom. It is one of the smallest molecules, atoms bound together, that exists naturally. And it exists everywhere! Water affects just about everything we do because this very special molecule can do some very special things that most molecules cannot.

1. Water is polar.

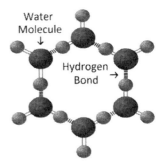

Water Molecule ↓

Hydrogen Bond →

What this means is that water molecules interact with other water molecules. Oxygen likes to borrow electrons from the hydrogen atoms in water. This makes the oxygen slightly more negative and the hydrogen slightly more positive. We all know the saying opposites attract. This is what happens with water. The oxygen of a water molecule attracts the hydrogen of another water molecule. This is called a hydrogen bond because only hydrogen can make this happen. With all of the molecules of water doing this they end up lining up in an ordered fashion.

40

2. Water is cohesive and adhesive.

Cohesion, when the molecules hold themselves together as a result of the hydrogen bonds, happens with water. Cohesion is why insects can walk on water without falling in. Water is also adhesive and 'sticks' to other molecules, due to the hydrogen bonds. This is particularly important with plants. Adhesion allows for water to move up, against gravity, in a plant by 'sticking' to the walls of the xylem. A similar thing happens in our circulatory and lymphatic systems.

3. Water has surface tension.

Surface tension is due to cohesion, water sticking to itself. This means that there is a force pulling the water molecules together, reducing the chance of other molecules from penetrating the barrier. Think of when you pour hot chocolate mix onto your water. For a short time it just sits on the surface of the water. We use a spoon to break the surface tension so the mixture will blend into the water. Soap commonly is what we use to break the surface tension of water when we need to break the bonds between water molecules. Try putting some oil on water then dropping a drop of liquid soap in the middle of the oil. The oil will quickly move to the edges of the bowl.

4. Water moderates temperature.

Water has the unique ability to absorb heat and hold onto it while changing its temperature only slightly. To understand this, you must know that heat is actually the energy that a molecule has that causes it to move, kinetic energy. The more kinetic energy something has, the more heat it produces, and therefore it has a higher temperature. When something has high enough heat/kinetic energy it will evaporate, changing from a liquid to a gas. Water specifically can absorb a lot of heat before it evaporates. This is easy to see with the transition from ice to water in melting. Water can hold so much heat that water can actually be colder than freezing and still be a liquid. Try freezing a bottle of water on its side and carefully remove it from the freezer when it is nearly frozen. When you then shift, stir, or shake this water it will immediately freeze with the kinetic energy you add to it.

5. Water is a universal solvent, almost.

When you need to dissolve something, water is an ideal substance to use. Not everything dissolves in water, but everything living uses water as it's solvent. This is why our blood is water based, why we drink water, why plants bring nutrient containing water up from their roots, and why everything we know as life is based on water. Nothing else even comes close to being as effective as water at dissolving things. When you dissolve a material in water, what is happening is that the molecules in the solid material, such as salt, separate from each other and are surrounded by water molecules, occupying the space between water molecules. This only happens with molecules that are hydrophilic, water loving, and does not happen with molecules that are hydrophobic (lipophilic, oil loving). This is important because this separation of water and oil is what makes our cells possible. Our cells are made of hollow balls of lipids (oil molecules) and all our cell parts are water soluble and fit inside of the ball of lipid molecules.

6. Water alters acid/base conditions.

Sometimes a hydrogen molecule will separate from the oxygen all together, leaving us with OH-, hydroxide. This separation and subsequent re-bonding to form H_2O again, are what gives us our pH scale. There is always free hydrogen floating around in a solution and depending on what other molecules are in the water, such as an acid there may be more or less free hydrogen. The more hydrogen that is not bonded on hydroxide, the more acidic a solution is, having a lower pH.

There is a constant binding and unbinding of free hydroxide and hydrogen depending on which needs to be borrowed by other molecules in the solution. Our bodies require different pH levels in different areas for different enzymes to work. Enzymes make sure that everything in our body is working properly from our digestion, our brain function, and even the growth of our nails.

WATER AND WELLNESS

Taking into consideration these properties of water, how does water really affect our wellness? Many of the properties are easiest to understand when thinking about plants and insects. It is challenging for us to view our own lives on such a small scale, to realize how individual droplets of water affect our lives.

For humans, the most important thing about water is its ability to balancing numbers of molecules through a membrane. It can do this because it is such a good solvent. Membranes allow some molecules to go through them and others are prevented, usually because they are too large. Membranes separate our individual cells from each other and from the outside world. In our bodies, our blood, which is basically water with stuff in it, circulates around. When there is an imbalance between the amount of dissolved material in the blood and the cell, the membrane will allow either the material, if small enough, or water to go through the membrane to try to balance the concentration inside and outside of the cell.

If you want to try an experiment on this, take a small cube of potato and soak one piece in water and another in a highly salted water. Weight them before and after and their weights should change. The piece in just water should gain some weight, because the water will be absorbed by the potato, trying to reduce the percentage of 'stuff' in its water to equal the plain water. The piece in salt water should lose some weight as the water from the potato moves into the salt water to try to reduce the concentration of salt in the water. While this is a very crude experiment, what is going on is the membrane is allowing a change in **osmotic balance**, the percentage of 'stuff' dissolved in water on each side of the membrane. Osmotic balance is very important in our bodies and is one of the main things we can directly experience when we are dehydrated and need more water.

This balance between the inside of cells and the outside of cells is also important in a few specific systems of our body. This is how we absorb nutrients in our digestive system, how we excrete toxins in our renal system, and how we are able to absorb and excrete things through our skin as well. Without having a proper amount of water, we are unable to absorb nutrients from our digestive system and we are unable to get rid of the toxins that have built up in our bodies through urination and sweating.

These processes are incredibly important. With all of the things we learned about food doing in our bodies, how could we possibly survive without getting all of the different kinds of nutrients our body's needs? What about toxins? In our bodies they can do major damage. They can stimulate gene transcription that we do not want, they can physically damage tissues, they can cause our bodies to have an immune response, and much more. We want to get rid of these toxins more than anything. Without a proper fluid balance in our bodies, we cannot do this.

Not only do we need water for the transportation of molecules in and out of our bodies, we also need water for the transportation in and out of cells. This is important because once nutrients are inside our bodies they need to get to the right cells through the blood. When we have enough water our blood is able to flow more freely, and is able to hold more nutrients for transportation.

In an individual cell level, blood offers oxygen and other nutrients that are dissolved in the blood to the cell. The cell can only accept them if the cell has a high enough water concentration and a low enough concentration of the molecules that they are accepting from the blood. Without this, water balance our cells would not be able to absorb nutrients. When our cells have more water, the spaces in the membrane that molecules can wiggle their way through are larger, and larger molecules can enter. This can be detrimental when there is inflammation. Larger, more damaging molecules, are able to pass through the membrane. This is important in both our digestive system and in the hydration of our skin, the places where we take nutrients into our bodies.

Not only is hydration important for this fluid balance, it has a few other uses that can be important. The first, joint lubrication, is what allows us to move. Most of our large joints, where two bones meet, have a joint capsule. This joint capsule is filled with a fluid that helps to nourish the bones, tendons, and ligaments all meeting there to support moving the joint. If this space was solid and not fluid the bones would not be able to move freely. Hydration specifically helps to lubricate our joints only when we are using the joints. When we use a joint that is 'stiff' or hasn't been used in a while there is an immune response that tells the body to send more fluid to the area. This fluid reduces pain in the moment and, with consistent use of the joint, the fluid will help heal and nourish the joint. This is one of the reasons that the main treatments for arthritis pain is to move the affected joint.

Hydration also specifically affects our mucous membranes. Anyone that has ever had a cold knows this. The more hydrated you are the thinner your mucous in in your nose is. This makes it much easier to blow our noses and remove more of the potentially infectious molecules in our noses. While we may not enjoy blowing our noses, it is best to be well hydrated so we can expel mucus through our noses. There are other mucous membranes in our bodies that are directly related to our hydration levels and they are all improved with higher hydration levels. Our mouths have their own mucous membranes and these are the easiest to see if we are hydrated or not. It takes about a week of being hydrated for your mouth mucous to be affected. If you spit when you talk or notice that you have stringy mucous in your mouth you are really dehydrated. This should be a sign that you need to double or triple your daily water intake.

If you feel thirsty it is already too late to drink water - you should still drink! Different systems take different amounts of time to be affected by your water intake. Your mucous membranes are affected about a week later for instance. Staying constantly hydrated will actually help reduce your likelihood of getting sick by keeping your mucous in your nose constantly flowing outward. Feeling thirsty is generally a result you experience a few days after when you were not getting enough water.

The most dramatic sign of dehydration is constant dry skin. While there are other causes to dry skin, this can show up to a month of dehydration and can take just as long to repair. There are many images of woman online who have started drinking high levels of water and have greatly improved the quality of their skin. It is true, and it works. You just need to always be drinking water. Your skin can also absorb water through creams and lotions but due to evaporation this is not a long-term solution for hydration. Skin helps keep moisture inside of your body but it does still evaporate. The more you are taking in the more hydrated your skin will be as it slowly allows moisture to evaporate.

WATER PATHWAY

Water has a very clear path in the body. It is swallowed, absorbed in the digestive tract, circulates the body in the blood, and absorbed by tissues and cells that need it. When it is not needed, it goes to the kidneys where it is used to pull out toxins into the kidneys and is then excreted in the form of urine. Water is not supposed to come out in your stool but sometimes it does. This can be because of two different things. Either you are not absorbing all of the water in your digestive tract or more water is being added to your bowels to moisten their mucosal membranes.

When you are hydrated enough, your bowels should be adequately moistened and your stool should be solid yet moist. When your stool becomes too watery and you experience diarrhea and is generally a sign that you are not absorbing the water you drink. Your body cannot excrete that much water into your bowels that fast. When your body is having a hard time absorbing water, such as when you are sick, adding electrolytes to your water will help adjust the osmotic balance and more water will be absorbed. We have all heard about giving children, who are sick with diarrhea, electrolytes. Electrolytes help the body to both absorb the water and nutrients that the body may be missing. Excess water in the stool reduces the absorption of nutrients in the digestive tract. Most adults do not have trouble with this but if you are struggling to absorb enough water in your digestive tract, adding a bit of salt, such as celtic sea salt to your water can increase the absorption. Celtic sea salt is not just normal table salt, it has extra nutrients and minerals that help you absorb more water. That does not mean sprinkle more salt on your French Fries.

As we touched on earlier, water is very important for getting rid of toxins in the body. You should not be afraid of going to the bathroom. If you are challenged by this, keep practicing. Having a healthy elimination and frequent urination is important. Some people are worried by high levels of urination. While this can be detrimental due to timing or location, it is important that we keep urinating regularly through the day. When properly hydrated, you should consider 8-10 a healthy number of urinations throughout the day. Yes, that is a lot but it depends on exercise, bladder size, and hydration level. Paying attention to the color of your urine is also important to know your hydration levels.

Your urine should be clear to a pale yellow when you are properly hydrated. If your urine is pale yellow, especially when diluted in the water of your toilet, you need to drink more water. The color or your urine is probably the best and fastest way to see your hydration level. The color changes depending on how many toxins are being excreted from your kidneys. The number of toxins is going to generally be the same and the amount of water that is excreted with the toxins will make the color lighter with more water. You can change the color or your urine with just one cup of water and affect the next time you urinate. Because of this, it is common to have darker urine first thing in the morning because you are not drinking water through the night while you sleep. Do not be worried about this. Just drink some water when you wake up.

Note: there are a variety of pharmaceuticals that can alter the color of your urine. If you notice a dramatic change, contact your doctor and discuss the change with them.

What are the signs you want to be aware of, to know your hydration level?

During the past 1-3 hours?

During the last day?

During the last 2-3 days?

During the last week?

During the last month?

Do you experience any of these signs?

Are you happy with your water intake? Why or why not?

What are you currently doing to increase your water intake?

How would your life improve if you were to increase your water intake?

Answers
Past 1-3 hours: color of urine

Last day: Moisture in stool, Number of urinations

Last 2-3 days: Dry mouth

Last week: Mucous stickiness, Joint pain

Last month: Skin dryness

CHAPTER 4: BEING CONSCIOUS OF OUR BODY

Homework Assignment 2

Observe and record the following for a week.

- What food do you eat?
- How much of each food?
- What time do you eat?
- Anything else that goes in your mouth: all drinks, cigarettes, gum and mints, medicines and supplements.

This chapter starts our focus on food and eating habits. First off - don't even think about the word 'diet.' It is a word that does not serve us in this day and age. Diet fads come and go but most often they are not long term methods of getting the nourishment you need. This is why I have started using the term 'conscious eating.'

Have you tried diets in the past? Which ones?

What kind of success did you have with your previous methods of eating?

Are you currently experiencing challenges with how you interact with food?

What does conscious eating mean to you?

> *Conscious eating is learning to pay attention to how different foods make your body feel so that you can adjust your eating to better your experience of your body.*

LISTENING TO YOUR BODY

The hardest part about practicing conscious eating is learning to pay attention to your body and how it feels. With diets you often spend most of your time hearing what other people say about your body and measuring yourself. Shouldn't it matter how you actually feel? It does take some practice to always pay attention to your own body so let's start with a simple check in.

Spend three minutes with one of your personal meditation practices to relax and center yourself. Listen to your body and see what it has to say. How do you feel right now? Create a list of words to describe how you are feeling.

Go back and look at those words. If you see a word describing an emotion, underline it. If you see a word that describes a physical sensation, one that could be described by the sense of touch, circle it. The words you have circled are the 'feeling' words that you are looking for.

This is not generally how we describe how our body feels and these are the words that will aid you in learning more about your body.

Go through the list below of how one may describe their body and do the same underlining and circling. Consider putting an X through the other words that are not true physical sensations or emotions.

sad	achy	hungry	tired
stuffed	tight	wet	gooey
hard	comfortable	fine	light
soft	depressed	happy	dry

This practice is one of the hardest things to do. We have to relearn how to listen to our bodies, and describe what we are experiencing with words that are physical feelings. Often we mistakenly label emotions as physical sensations, like achy and comfortable. You cannot touch a book and say "This feels achy." You can touch a book and say "This feels hard." By practicing with your feeling words you will start to experience a closer relationship between your mental state and how your body works. Let's practice. Try to stick to using physical sensation words only.

How are your legs feeling right now?

How does your waist region feel right now?

How does your abdomen feel right now?

How do your arms feel right now?

How does your chest feel right now?

How does your neck region feel right now?

How does your head feel right now?

Listening is always a challenge. When we have things on our mind, are stressed, busy with work and family obligations, we forget to pay attention to our bodies and listen. Practice is what can really help to make listening a habit. Keep practicing. To begin your practice at paying attention to your body, spend this week recording what food goes into your body.

Probably your hardest assignment in this book will be to keep a food log. For this include approximate quantities and list everything you put into your mouth, including drinks, supplements, and medications. This will get you started in observing what you are putting into your body. Try to not alter what you are eating this month, just observe. You can also create a tick box for each cup of water, serving of fruits or vegetables, dairy products, coffee or tea, and tablespoon of oil. Label what each row refers to as to suit your needs.

CHAPTER 5: HYDRATION TECHNIQUES

Homework Assignment 3

Choose one of the hydration techniques from this chapter and choose to follow it for a week. Record in your journal what worked well for you and what challenged you with the hydration technique. Numbers 1, 2, 3, and 4 are recommended.

Now that we know a little more about what water is doing in our body and how to see if we are hydrated, let's talk about how to increase our hydration.

What steps are you currently taking to increase your hydration?

Are you able to do these things consistently and are you noticing a reduction in dehydration symptoms?

What is challenging you about increasing the amount of water you are drinking?

Here are a few techniques you can use to increase your water intake:

1. Every time you drink a cup of something that is not just water, drink a cup of water with it.

This helps to balance water intake with other types of fluids. Drinking water in this fashion can only increase your water intake over time, encouraging hydration.

2. Every time you urinate, drink a cup of water afterwards.

This is my favorite recommendation. The reason for this is because urination removes water from your body and when you immediately replenish this your body will immediately have more water for its needs. Most of the time we do not urinate a full 8oz cup of liquid so I always use this technique to slowly increase my hydration level when I am feeling dehydrated. This is a good tool to have because it does not stress my body out in trying to drink more.

3. Before you go to sleep, drink a cup of water.

While we sleep we do not have the ability to drink water. This is really important because some people will wake up in the night thirsty. By drinking water ahead of time you will reduce this. It is also an 8-hour period where we do not generally drink. Sometimes we will sweat while we sleep and we cannot replace this fluid. While unconscious, we use our time asleep to heal our bodies and we need water to be able to do this. Our detoxification process and kidneys are working while we are sleeping and we need water for them as well. Help all of these processes work better by drinking a cup of water before bed. Some people don't like to do this because they are worried they will wake up in the night to go to the bathroom. I truly believe that it is more important to drink the water and wake up to go to the bathroom, even if it happens multiple times. There are techniques in our sleep chapter to support you in getting back to sleep.

4.   When you wake up, drink a cup of water.

After all of our body's work while we are asleep it is important to re-hydrate it afterwards. It is common to urinate when you first wake up and if your urine is yellow it is even more important that you hydrate. If you are not urinating when you first wake up, you should drink more water through the day. It means you were not hydrated enough when you went to bed.

5.   For every 30 minutes of exercise you do, drink a cup of water afterwards.

You sweat when you exercise and you need to replenish this water just like when you urinate. If you are seeing a personal trainer regularly they can determine the exact amount of water you should intake after exercise. As a general rule 8oz, one cup, per 30 minutes of moderate to high intensity exercise is a good level.

6.   Always have a water bottle with you.

You are not going to drink water if you don't have it available to you. When you have a water bottle sitting next to you every day, you are going to actually see it every so often and drink from it. Use the water bottle as a way to check in with yourself. Are you feeling thirsty? Yes? Finish that water bottle and go get some more because you are dehydrated. No? Drink ½ a cup every hour through the day and you will maintain your hydration.

7. Buy a fancy glass that you can use just for water.

When at home or in the office, you will love drinking water when you get to use your fancy glass. I have a special clear glass water bottle and a beautiful glass that I keep with me and in my kitchen. When I see the glass I want to use it because it is special so I drink a glass of water. It is nice to feel fancy every so often. So splurge on a nice glass to use and you will enjoy it even more. Been eying that cocktail glass at the store but don't make cocktails at home? Get it, and use it to drink water out of. Feeling fancy may make you enjoy drinking water.

8. Have a water filter.

Having good quality water is important to drink too. We don't want to be drinking water that is not filtered, containing who knows what, prescription medications, fluoride, and other things added to the water. Buying spring water or having a general filter is ideal. DO NOT DRINK DI WATER. You may see this in stores and think "oh that looks like it is the best. It is completely filtered." This is not drinking water. DI water, which is deionized, is pure H2O and does not contain the natural minerals we need from water. It can actually dehydrate you to drink DI water. If you have a reverse osmosis water filter at home, go for it, but make sure you are adding minerals back in or you will be having the same challenge as the DI water.

When choosing your water source, keep the environment in mind. Purchasing disposable bottles of water, while convenient, has its costs that we generally cannot see. Keep in mind the fossil fuel expenditure needed to make each bottle and the damage of the plastics themselves. These reasons make filers a much better option for your home and the earth.

Of these techniques, which ones would serve you to incorporate into your life? Make a plan now, on how you will use these techniques to increase your hydration.

CHAPTER 6: MOVEMENT PRACTICES

Homework Assignment 4

Do you have a water bottle yet? Keep it filled all week and no more than 10 feet from you at all times. Having it available makes all the difference.

Track how many minutes of movement you do every day until you hit 30 minutes for 5 days in a row. This is any kind of movement and can include things like standing and doing dishes.

Exercising can be a challenge, but the take home message from this section is that any movement is better than no movement, and that lack of movement can be more detrimental than you think. Make it fun and you won't need to worry!

We all could probably use more movement in our lives and we all know it. Getting a regular movement and exercise schedule in your life is probably the single hardest thing you will ever do. There are so many different ways to increase your movement and we all have good reason to do so. While I chose dancing most frequently, I dance for the enjoyment I get out of it. It is also a great way to socialize, exercise, reduce stress, and oddly, it helps keep me hydrated as I drink more often when dancing. Your choice of exercise may be different than this, and that is wonderful!

Let us briefly overview some benefits to movement. We all know that exercise is most commonly suggested for weight management through increased metabolism. Exercise increases your bodies metabolic function. What does that mean? Metabolism is the process by which we gain energy from our food to run all of the systems in our bodies. Each cell also has metabolic functions that help run the cell. By exercising we are increasing our energy needs so our body needs to compensate by digesting more efficiently. When we are exercising to gain strength and flexibility we slightly damage and push our muscles to their extremes which slightly damages the tissues. The healing process can be thought of as the strengthening of our muscles. So we have to heal our tissues after exercise and we have to digest more efficiently to have the proteins to heal damaged tissues.

We all have different reasons to include movement in our lives. For most it is because they feel they have to exercise because their doctors told them they should. This is not a reason that will motivate you long term into moving. Think back to why you want to increase movement in your life. For some people it is out of fear because they have family history of cardiovascular or heart disease. They want to stay around longer to support and love their families. Others use exercise as a stress reducer. Exercise is great at reducing stress and feeling good is a real reason people can stick with movement long term.

Why do you want to include more movement in your life?

What kinds of movement have you done in the past? Did you enjoy it?

What kinds of movement are you including in your life right now?

Commonly, we don't turn to exercise and movement until we are already ill, or we realize we have risk factors for an illness that could be reduced through exercising. Exercise and movement can also help prevent many common illnesses primarily by strengthening many of the body's systems, so they are less likely to become injured or infected. Exercise improves your musculoskeletal system, cardiovascular system, respiratory system, immune system, digestive system, stress response, and lymphatic and detoxification systems.

Pain commonly will scare people away from exercise. It hurts at first and can be dangerous if you are not properly supervised when you are not used to exercising. When you are starting to add more movement in to your life it is important that you do it safely. If you have any questions on what you feel is appropriate movement, please seek a medical professional. And I am not just saying this. Go talk to your doctor about it.

To begin this, let's start with a simple questionnaire to see if you are healthy enough to begin or continue exercise. (American College of Sports Medicine 2015 Guidelines for aerobic exercise participation.)

Do you already participate in regular exercise? If yes, give yourself one point.

Give yourself two points if you have a known cardiovascular, metabolic, or renal disease such as hypertension, diabetes, or others.

Give yourself two point if you answer yes to any of the following:

- Has your doctor ever said that you have a heart condition <u>and</u> that you should only do physical activity that is recommended by a doctor?
- Do you feel pain in your chest when you do physical activity?
- In the past month, have you had chest pain when you were not doing physical activity?

- Do you lose your balance because of dizziness or do you ever lose consciousness?
- Do you have a bone or joint problem (for example, back, knee, or hip) that could be made worse by a change in your physical activity?
- Is your doctor currently prescribing drugs (for example, water pills) for your blood pressure or heart condition?

Results

0 Points   Congratulations! You can start exercising!

1 Point   Congratulations! You can continue exercising!

2-4 Points   It is recommended that you get clearance by your doctor before beginning to exercise. If you already exercise, you may continue to exercise at a moderate intensity level. Seek out clearance from a doctor before doing vigorous exercise.

5 Points   Discontinue exercise and seek medical clearance

Moderate intensity physical activity is defined for this as the ability to speak while exercising but not sing.

Vigorous intensity physical activity is defined as activity when you are unable to talk while exercising.

GENERAL FITNESS RECOMMENDATIONS

The Centers for Disease Control and Prevention (CDC) and American College of Sports Medicine (ACSM) jointly recommend that:

> *'Every US adult should accumulate over the course of the day, 30 minutes or more of moderate intensity physical activity on most, preferably all days of the week.'*

The American Heart Association (AHA) 2007 guidelines recommend all healthy adults under age 55 have a minimum of 30 minutes a day of moderate aerobic exercise, 5 days a week, or high intensity aerobic exercise 20 minutes per day, 3 days a week. What makes exercise moderate or intense? There is some math you can do but generally, moderate heart rate is when you are doing an exercise and you are able to talk but not able to sing. When you reach your high intensity heart rate you are no longer able to talk. A low intensity heart rate you are able to sing.

There are many online applications that will help you find your heart rate ranges, but even these numbers will be different for every individual depending on their resting heart rate and their age. For some individuals that are less fit, and have a higher resting heart rate, it can be very easy to reach moderate intensity exercise. On the other hand, for very fit individuals with a lower resting heart rate it can be extremely difficult to get your heart rate up for high intensity exercise. This is great news for you if you are only starting to add more movement to your life. It is going to be easier for you than someone who is already doing movement to get the same benefits.

KINDS OF MOVEMENT

When many people are told to exercise, they think their only option is to run. There are so many other kinds of movement and they all offer different kinds of benefits to the individual. Let's start by breaking down the three different kinds of exercise: cardio, stretching, and strengthening.

Cardio

This is what most people think about when they think about exercise. Cardio is the exercise that is most effective at getting your heart rate up. This kind of work is labeled cardio because it encourages our cardiovascular system to work harder. These kinds of activities include running, climbing stairs, dancing, boxing, most team sports, and swimming.

The benefits from cardio exercise generally focus around strengthening your heart muscle, creating endurance in your skeletal muscles, and improving your lung capacity and strength. Cardio can improve your lymphatic flow to detoxify your body. It can reduce your stress responses by releasing molecules related to pleasure. Generally, when doing cardio workouts, because your body is focused on supplying oxygen to your muscles rather than digesting food you do not increase your digestion. However, when doing certain kinds of movements around your waist it can support peristaltic movement through your intestines so that food can move through more effectively.

What would you enjoy doing the most for cardio activity?

Of the benefits to cardio exercise, which ones do you think would most support your personal wellbeing?

What would actually encourage you to add more cardio exercise into your life?

Adding cardio exercise was the hardest of these for me. Having been a dancer, I often will participate in social dance. I found I was not hitting my moderate heart rate however. I am not in great cardiovascular health, so when I then set out to try jogging it was not an option with my asthma. I began doing more invigorating waking, similar to speed walking. What has kept me going on this was listening to audio books. If I want to continue in the story I need to walk. This was excellent encouragement for me to actually get more cardio exercise in my life.

That sounds like everything we need to do for exercise right? As long as we can run, jump, breathe, and circulate our blood and food we are good. Maybe not. Though it may not seem important to you now, if you want to be able to be as active and capable of doing your everyday activities well into your years you should start increasing your strength and flexibility now.

Strengthening

Strengthening, or strength training, exercises are ones we are familiar with, but we don't generally understand how they can be beneficial to us. Cardio exercises strengthen our hearts. Other strengthening exercises focus on our skeletal muscles. Having strong muscles are important to our everyday activities such as carrying items like boxes and groceries, standing for long periods of time, and caring for your family.

Strengthening activities usually require weight bearing activities such as using free weights, weight machines, or body weight. If you are not a member of a gym it can be difficult to have access to weight machines. Free weights are helpful to have but not necessary for strengthening the body. Your own body weight works very effectively to strengthen its muscles. This is the principal of Pilates; your own body is heavy enough to provide significant benefit when you move your body in opposition to gravity. For individuals just starting out adding more movement to their lives, standing up can itself be a strengthening exercise. If your muscles are not used to holding your body upright, it can cause strain on your body to just stand. Practice doing your normal desk work, standing up, to start this kind of strengthening.

To strengthen a muscle group, you contract the muscle, shorten it, and either hold it or repeatedly contract and release it over time. Contracting repeatedly, or holding a contraction for a period of time, damages the contracting protein molecules in the muscle. As these molecules repair themselves they become stronger. You cannot strengthen your muscles without using them, causing microscopic damage first.

Have you previously done any strengthening activities? What activities?

What do you do in your daily life where you would benefit from being stronger?

What has stopped you in the past from doing more strengthening activities?

Strengthening exercises also happen throughout our daily life and are not always necessary to meet daily needs. If you notice that you are unable to, or are challenged by, regular activities, you may want to try to do strengthening activities more frequently to improve your ability. Increasing your abilities is the goal of strengthening exercises.

I have had challenges with strengthening activities. With the social dance I do, my right and left sides of my body are not always the same strength. I then choose to carry my bags in my other arm and initiate going up stairs on my other leg to try to balance the strength on the two sides of my body. The most effective thing I have done was carrying a water bottle while walking so my right arm could get stronger by adding a bit more weight to it.

STRETCHING

Many people don't like to stretch. When you do cardio it will sometimes hurt the next day. Same with strengthening exercises. It is much harder with stretching because it feels uncomfortable while you are doing it. When I teach kids to stretch it is a very odd battle. Our bodies say "this hurts" when it really does not. It feels uncomfortable, unfamiliar to our muscles, so we naturally do not want to stretch. I tell the kids, "it is a good kind of hurt and the more you do it the less it will hurt and the better your whole body will feel." We all know this to be true innately. When you just have to yawn to stretch your jaw, stand up after sitting for a long period of time, arch your back, or stretch your arms and wrists after typing these are all examples of stretches your body wants through the day.

Have you previously done any stretching activities? What muscle groups?

What do you do in your daily life where you would benefit from being more flexible?

What has stopped you in the past from doing more stretching?

Stretching primarily increases flexibility, the length your muscles can expand to when relaxed. To understand this, think about your quadriceps, on the front of your thigh, and your hamstrings, on the back of your thigh. When you stand up straight and bend forward at the waist you stretch your hamstrings, they get longer, and your quadriceps, contract, get shorter. The reverse is the case when you lift your leg behind you, your hamstrings get shorter, contract, and your quadriceps get longer and stretch.

This opposition of stretching and contracting happens over almost all of the joints in your body. Other easy examples you can try out are in your forearm, ankles, neck, and your knees. Because of this opposition, whenever you strengthen a muscle group, you have to also stretch it so the opposing muscle group also gets to be strengthened and stretched. One way to visualize why oppositional training is necessary is to think about how many athletes walk, arms pulled out to their sides and bent at the elbows and a wide stance. This posture is due to over working the biceps in the arms, without equally working the triceps behind the arm and not stretching the biceps. The legs are wide because of a focus on strengthening the quadriceps without stretching them and strengthening the hamstrings.

But why do we need to stretch? These athletes may have a stiff walk but they don't seem to have any problems. They exercise after all.

Having done a lot of stretching with dance growing up, I always have a desire to do it. Finding a way to causally stretch is hard. Even when I have a chance to go on a walk and stop to stretch, others who are walking joke with me in a way that implies the situation is not 'normal.' Stretching is something that even the exercise community struggles with including regularly. My favorite way to get more stretching is doing it while watching television and relaxing.

But do we really need to do all of these things? As we age, we need to have stronger muscles to hold our bodies upright. Think of the old man or woman, stooped over as they go about their day. They became stooped by not strengthening their back and neck muscles. They cannot fully extend their arms to reach the shelves that are at their shoulder height. They have trouble bending over to tie their shoes. While some of these may be unavoidable, proper stretching and strengthening can greatly reduce the likelihood of these occurring and being irreversible. Even now, do you struggle to lift heavy boxes, do your muscles ache from going upstairs, do you have a hard time standing up for thirty or more minutes? All of these things that we do through our day are directly related to our strength, flexibility, and how they interact with each other.

MOVEMENT PRACTICE STAGE 1

I haven't done much exercise before/I am just starting to exercise/I am new to adding movement to my life

I am glad you are starting on this path to increase movement in your life. Do not feel discouraged if you are not ready to begin yet. Adding movement to your life is one of the hardest yet most rewarding things you can do for yourself. Don't give up. You can do anything you put your mind to, even if it takes some time.

If you have been cleared by your doctor to start movement and exercise, the best place to start is simply walking. Now walking does not count as moderate activity towards your 3-thirty minute sessions a week but it will take some time until you will get there. If you are able to walk around your neighborhood, starting by walking for even five minutes is good. If you can walk for five minutes, reach for ten, and so on. If you can do five but not ten minutes of walking, try to do five minutes of walking twice a day. Continue to increase in this kind of progression until you are able to walk for 30 minutes a day.

The practice for this chapter may be challenging when it is cold outside but walking around your home is just as effective. If you work in an office space or similar, sitting most of the day, standing up every 15 minutes can be helpful. If you remember from chapter 1, we mentioned that sitting can be more detrimental to your health than anything else. Remember to just stand up and walk around for 5 minutes or so every hour and this is a great way to make sure you start getting movement while at work. This is also an excellent time to start simple stretches and wiggling.

I love telling people to wiggle. It's great! Wiggling, when you don't do much movement, is great. It helps to loosen up joints that may be stiff. It prompts you to move your body in a way you may not be used to, engaging different muscles without too much force. It also gets the blood moving and lymph circulating similar to cardio activities without a large increase in heart rate.

Lymph circulation helps to detoxify the body. As our blood circulates through our body, it can sometimes leak waste into our tissues. The lymph nodes collect this waste and the lymphatic circulation drains it back into the blood to be removed from the body. This circulatory system does not have muscles to push the toxins along. The only way to move this waste back into your blood is to move your body and the muscles surrounding the lymph tissues.

If you are worried about the idea of wiggling around in your work place or home, the shower is a great place to wiggle around, providing you do it carefully. One great practice in the shower is to make sure you have cleaned your entire body without any back washers or similar to extend your reach. This kind of movement, reaching to clean your whole body, forces you to move around in the same ways you are not used to, the same as wiggling. Try it!

Now, if you have already started this kind of simple movement daily, don't stop! When starting a new practice a few things can happen. If you get through 4 days and skip a day it can be hard to go back the next day. Having read our chapter on behavior change, you have seen how consistency in creating a new habit or lifestyle is key. Even if you reduce your time moving on that 5th day, that is much better than not practicing your new lifestyle addition.

CHAPTER 7: BREATHING AND MEDITATION TECHNIQUES

Homework Assignment 5

Observe and record the following for a week as you practice breathing and meditation for sleep support.

- When do you start getting ready for bed?
- When do you get into bed?
- What time do you fall asleep?
- What time do you wake up?
- What time you got out of bed?
- How many times did you wake up during the night that you remember?
- How long were you awake when you were up in the middle of the night?

When you were a kid, you probably heard someone talking about counting sheep to help you get to sleep. This idea is not new and many techniques of calming the mind are based on the same idea of organizing your thoughts into a mindless state. Meditation is one practice that can help to calm the mind. Another is practicing breathing, a common piece of meditation practices. One of the reasons that breathing is a great tool to use to support falling asleep is that as we increase our oxygen supply, our body systems relax. This is why anesthesia gas often contains a high concentration of oxygen.

Breathing Technique 1:

Rhythmic breathing is key to most breathing techniques. This rhythm, something that is regular and slow, can be hard to develop. It is important to start with simple techniques if you do not have experience paying attention to your breath. Spend some time just paying attention and observing your breathing, if this is not something you have done previously, before you start to alter your normal breathing patterns.

Observe how long it takes you to take a breath. Do you breathe in for longer than you breathe out?

What parts of your body move when you breathe?

Are there any sounds you hear, or anything you feel, when you breathe?

Do you pause between breathing in and out, or back in again?

After you have spent a few minutes observing your breath start adjusting your breathing so that it is more regular. I suggest first starting with an easy counting method. Breathe in 1, 2, 3, 4 and then breathe out 1, 2, 3, 4. Count regular and slow. The slower you count the harder it will be. If you feel yourself struggling to breathe at the speed you are counting, speed up your counting a bit. Try to stretch out your breathing to get a more full breath of air.

Practice this technique daily for about 10 minutes. When I was first practicing conscious breathing, I found that playing music while I practiced served me. This was because I could practice keeping time to the music while breathing, counting the music. I had to search for a few songs to find one that fit a breathing pace that encouraged a longer breath than my natural breath, but was still comfortable for me. After about two weeks of daily practice, this breathing practice should become easy, and you can start challenging yourself with additional techniques. Continue to return to this practice to begin all of your breathing practice sessions.

Breathing Technique 2:

Learning how to do a full breath can be difficult. It is best to practice this lying down with your knees bent and touching with your hands on your stomach. To start, observe how you are already breathing, using the same check in from the first technique. Pay attention to how your hands feel on your stomach. Are they moving? Pay attention to your hands and as you breathe in and allow your stomach to rise, and fall as you breathe out. Over time, practicing this for a few minutes each night will help you to increase your lung capacity.

When you have become familiar with breathing through your stomach this way, return to focusing on your breathing while sitting up. To learn how to use your lungs most effectively you will need to have space for your body to expand in all directions. Return to practicing your 1-4 counting pattern of breathing. Breathe in 1: expand air into your stomach, 2: breathing in air to you rib cage, 3-4: breathe air into your chest, upper lobes of your lungs, and back. Reverse. Breathe out 1 from the air in your chest, 2: from the air in your rib cage, 3: with the air from your stomach, and 4: releasing your muscles and expelling the remaining air from your lungs.

This full breath takes a long time to master. The reason we focus on breathing from the belly first is because so much of what we observe growing up, and how we are conditioned to breathe, is breathing from the chest, a very shallow type of breath. This deeper method of breathing supports using our entire lung capacity, strengthening all of our muscles associated with breathing, and even supports lymphatic flow to detoxify our bodies. Strengthening our muscles to breathe can be very important if you experience asthma attacks, shortness of breath, anxiety attacks, or if you are new to higher levels of movement and exercise. Increasing your cardio activity can be as simple as starting by improving the quality and strength of your breath. Breathing in full breaths is one piece that is important with both Yoga and Pilates practices.

Breathing Technique 3:

The third technique I will talk about will probably only come once you have increased your lung capacity through many months of practicing breathing technique 2. This next level of meditative breathing is called box breathing. The main purpose of practicing this breathing is to slow your breath even further. Slowing your breath also slows your pulse, slows your mind, and allows you to relax. Like the other breathing techniques to receive the relaxation benefits you need to practice this until it becomes second nature to breathe with this pattern.

To do this technique you will again be counting and for this example we will continue with our count of 4. Breathe in 1, 2, 3, 4; hold your breath 1, 2, 3, 4; breathe out 1, 2, 3, 4; hold your breath out 1, 2, 3, 4. This is very hard to do. You can picture a box while you do this to remember where in the sequence you are. Moving up the side of a box to breathe in and increasing the air in your lungs, hold it on the flat top of the box, breathe out moving down and lowering the amount of air in your lungs, and holding the emptiness in your lungs along the bottom of the box.

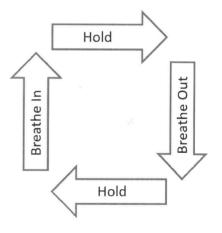

If you start with using the number 4 to count to you have already reduced the number of breaths you will take in a minute down to 4. Most adults take between 5-6 breaths a minute. Over time you can increase the number you use and you will be able to slow your breathing even more. If you have even a 6-count box breath you have slowed your breathing down to 2.5 breaths a minute. With breathing this slow it is important to make sure you are taking the full breaths you learned how to with technique 2. This is not a breathing technique for daily use but rather one that can be used to center and calm yourself. This makes it ideal to practice before bed.

These three breathing techniques can be very beneficial in relaxing and centering your body and mind while trying to sleep. They can also serve in meditation, and for stress relief at any time. As you become more skilled in controlling your breath, you may notice you want to meditate to become more aware of your body. This is an excellent tool to use for stress reduction and in helping you to fall asleep. There are many resources for meditation and to start you out I have included two simple practices here. You may want to record your own voice reading some of this, to help guide you each time you practice one of these techniques.

MEDITATION TECHNIQUE: BODY CHECK-IN

Find a comfortable place to lie down. Make sure your back is straight and your head is supported by a small pillow. Insure that your pillow does not crunch your chin to your chest but elongates your neck. Relax your neck and shoulders letting your arms relax to your sides. Either relax your legs flat, or bend them with your feet flat on the floor and your knees resting against each other. Close your eyes.

Start by practicing your breathing techniques for a few minutes. Are you making full complete breaths? Breathe in through your nose, filling your lungs completely and fully expanding your stomach. Relax your shoulders as you breathe out, pushing air out with your stomach, fully releasing the air. Continue with your complete breathing, letting your body relax, and let go of any tension you are holding in your body.

When you are feeling relaxed, centered in your body, and thoughts are starting to pass you by, begin to focus on your feet. At your feet, clench them tightly. If you cannot, just think about tightening them up. Hold it! And release quickly. They should feel more relaxed than before you clenched them. Move to your ankles, clench them tightly. Hold. And release. Move slowly up your body in small increments focusing intently on specific parts of your body. Tighten them and release them. You can even start with individual toes. I recommend the following progression:

1. Feet	5. Upper Leg	9. Chest	13. Hands
2. Ankles	6. Waist	10. Shoulders	14. Face
3. Lower Leg	7. Stomach	11. Neck	15. Forehead
4. Knee	8. Back	12. Arms	16. Whole Body

Once you have relaxed your whole body, allow your body to rest in this state. Feel your body sink down into the floor. Feel the floor supporting your body and lifting you up as all of your muscles relax. Feel all of the tension you have been holding onto disappear as your body is present in a state of relaxation. Relax like this for a few minutes up to fifteen minutes, as time allows.

When you are ready, start to come out of your meditation and relaxed state. Start by bringing your attention to your finger tips and toes. Begin to wiggle them slowly and rock your head from side to side to waken up your senses. Open and close your hands, roll your ankles, and start to move some of the larger joints in your body. Take your time and do not sit right up or you may be a little light headed. Slowly roll onto your side and use your hands to support you as you start to sit up. If at any time you feel light headed lie back down on your side for a minute.

For some of us this may be uncomfortable the first few times we do this, or you may even fall asleep. While it can be a great technique for getting to sleep, this body review will help you to target where you hold your stress in your body, and help you to release all of the stress you experience in your body. Keep practicing until you can go through the whole sequence without falling asleep.

Feel free to adjust the sequence to your own needs and experiences of the practice. For example, I always feel tension in my back from exercise. When I focus on relaxing those muscles it causes me great discomfort. For this reason, I will occasionally skip that one if I think it will cause me too much discomfort. With the rest of my body relaxing, my back will then succumb and start to release through the remainder of the meditation practice.

MEDITATION TECHNIQUE: WALK THROUGH YOUR DAY

This meditation is good to do at the end of the day to let go of worries that have come up throughout the day. This meditation helps you break down any upsets and generate positive feelings about your experiences. Find a comfortable place to sit on a cushion with your legs crossed, or on a straight back chair where you can let your feet rest flat on the ground. Sit with your back straight, watching your hips to make sure they do not rock backwards, causing arching your back. Relax your shoulders, close your eyes, and begin to focus on your breath.

Are you making full complete breaths? Breathe in through your nose, filling your lungs completely and fully expanding your stomach. Relax your shoulders as you breathe out, pushing air out with your stomach, fully releasing the air. Continue with your complete breaths, letting your body relax and let go of any tension you are holding in your body.

When you are feeling relaxed, centered in your body, and thoughts are starting to pass you by, begin to focus on how you felt when you first woke up this morning, before you even got out of bed. Were you calm, relaxed, and ready to greet the morning? Were you angry at your alarm for going off and stressed about a meeting you have in an hour? If it was a negative feeling, calmly allow yourself to let go of that. You do not need to hold onto your upset. It is optional for you to feel that way. Tomorrow morning you will not need that feeling. Release any anger you may feel towards your emotions. If you have experienced a happy, positive waking up experience, remember that feeling. Let it fill your body with joy and appreciation for life at the start of each day.

Remember yourself getting up out of bed, starting your day. Did you go to the kitchen and make yourself breakfast? Did you go to the bathroom and shower? What were the next few things you did this morning? How did you feel when doing them? Neutral, bored, tired, anxious, pleasant? If you felt negative emotions, practice releasing those feelings. You do not need to hold onto them. They do not need to control you. You have control over your emotions, to choose if you want to be upset or not. Do you remember a time where you were happy while doing your morning routine? What did it feel like to you? What was causing you to be happy? Remember that feeling, and let it fill your body with joy and contentment.

After your morning routine, did you go to work, start playing with your children, head off to school, relax on the couch? Where did your day lead you next? How did you feel at this time? Release any negative feelings. You are stronger than them, and you have the right to feel good. Remember how you feel during this part of the day when you are having a good day. Are you smiling? Smile and bring in happy thoughts to associate with these actions you do on a daily basis.

Continue to think about how you experience your lunch time. Release your negative energies and allow positive thoughts and experiences to fill you. How do you experience your afternoon? As we begin to tire through the day it can be more difficult to focus on happy energies. Remember those happy experiences from your past and associate them with the new experiences you have in the afternoon. Did you have a confrontation? Spend some time releasing any anger and upset you experienced during this time. You do not need to hold onto it. Letting go of the upset is the first step in resolving the confrontation. Remember that the others involved in the confrontation are feeling just as bad as you. Everyone wants to experience joy and happiness. It is a universal truth. Releasing your upset will allow you to do this and also support others around you towards this goal.

How did you feel when you left work, picked up your kids, when your family came home, and your other afternoon and evening activities began? Did you experience any new upsets? Did you become frustrated because you or someone else was late? Did you forget to do something you meant to? Were upsets from earlier in the day still with you? Can you release these upsets so they do not interfere with your evening? Breathe deeply in and as you breathe out, release these upsets that you have not released from earlier in the day. You do not need them to be a healthy and happy individual. They do not need to control you. You have the choice to be happy and to release upsets you are carrying with you. Breathe in joy and contentment. Breathe out your upsets.

Think now to your evening activities, dinner, family time, catching up on work, and relaxing activities. Was your evening relaxing? Did you have fun, socialize or spend time alone? Was there anything that caused you anxiety, worry, stress, anger, or any other upset through your evening? Bring this upset to the front of your mind and let it go, pushing it out from your mind so you can bring forward pleasant thoughts about enjoying your evening. Let yourself smile, thinking about happy evenings you have experienced. Remember the happy experiences from last night. Let them fill you up so you associate the evening with happiness.

Remember yourself getting ready for bed and getting into bed for the night. Had you let go of all of your worries from the whole day or were things still being held onto? Were worries flying through your head as you tried to sleep or did you fall asleep quickly and peacefully? Release those worries as you have released the others from your day. Imagine yourself falling asleep peacefully and easily, with no worries from your day. Breathe in slowly and breathe out. And as you imagine yourself drifting into an imaginary sleep, begin to bring your awareness back to the present, the room you are in and the feeling of your body on your chair or cushion. Slowly rock back and forth to bring your thoughts back into your body. When you are ready, open your eyes.

MEDITATION RESOURCES

There are many free resources for meditations available. Searching on your smart phone for apps for guided meditations is excellent. These free audio lessons will walk you through meditations and guide your mind to think about certain topics for relaxation and stress reduction, as well as learning ways to calmly interact with people through viewing them in different lights. A favorite application of mine is Stop, Breathe, & Think. This application has goals that encourage you to try different meditations, at different times, and for different consistencies through your life. Can you reach the ultimate goal in this app, to meditate for 30 days in a row? You can do it!

There are also many great resources online for free guided meditations. Here are a few websites I enjoy.

- The Chopra Center
  http://www.chopra.com/ccl/guided-meditations

- UCLA Mindful Awareness Research Center
  http://marc.ucla.edu/body.cfm?id=22
- Fragrant Heart Meditation Center
  http://www.fragrantheart.com/

Meditations can focus on a certain challenge you are experiencing or they can just focus on your own wellbeing. Cater your meditation experience to your needs. The more you practice meditating the easier it will be and the more benefits you will experience. Keep at it and you will soon notice benefits from spending even five minutes a day in meditation.

While meditating and other mental wellness practices can be beneficial, some of us have challenges that are well beyond the scope of this. For challenges that threaten the safety of yourself or others, seek professional guidance **at once** from appropriate sources such as psychiatrists or law enforcement agencies depending on the situation.

A few good web resources are:

- Find a Psychiatrist
  http://psychiatrists.psychologytoday.com/rms/
- Depression Information
  http://www.helpguide.org/topics/depression.htm
- Help Hotlines
  http://www.teenhealthandwellness.com/static/hotlines
  While this site is geared towards teens, it offers many additional help lines for all ages including hotlines for domestic violence, homelessness, drug abuse, stress, and suicide.

CHAPTER 8: RELATIONSHIP WITH THE SELF

Homework Assignment 6

For a week you will spend time preparing for bed. To make sure you do this practice well, give yourself two hours before bed with no work and no screens - television, computer, phone, or otherwise. Take this time to read, meditate, take a bath, shower, enjoy a dessert or beverage, prepare clothes and supplies for the next day. Start to turn the lights off around your home so you can enjoy the dim light of the evening. Take two hours to relax. Continue to record the same journal. This may be really hard to find the time to do for most of us, especially if you have kids, because they require attention. You can make this a family time but it is important to make sure it is understood to be relaxation time, not running around time. This is an experiment to observe how your body experiences sleep with extra 'me time' prior to sleep.

I have put together a brief guide here to help support your spiritual side. Please take it with a grain of salt, knowing that what I offer is all about finding what serves you best in the place you are currently at in your life. Please accept that this may change over time and you may need to re-evaluate your spiritual beliefs and practices. This is one thing that I feel is important for your wellness in this area. Do not try to conform to the beliefs of others. Pay attention to your own beliefs and find the practices that best fit into your personal system.

Here I have included questions to get you thinking and to feel inspired, as that is the most important piece of spiritual engagement for your own wellness. Inspiration does not need to come in the form of motivation. It can come in the form of comfort and stability as well. A place and experience that makes you feel whole and wholly yourself. An experience that makes you feel proud to be who you are in the world, so that you can be fully present and share your gifts with others in a way that serves both you and them.

This is divided into three sections throughout this book. How you engage with yourself, others, and what we will label here as divine or spirit. This chapter's discussions will get you thinking more than the other chapters, as it is meant to. Use this time to explore your relationship with the world so that your interactions best serve who you are.

If you have a desire to jump further ahead and work on your connection with a religion, I recommend visiting BeliefNet.com and taking their Belief-O-Matic Quiz. You can find this at:
http://www.beliefnet.com/Entertainment/Quizzes/BeliefOMatic.aspx
When you provide your e-mail at the end of the quiz you will get a break down of all of the different religious paths your personal beliefs line up with. I am a large proponent of picking a religion based off of your beliefs. Do not try to conform your beliefs based on a predisposed religion. This asks hard questions, so consider this tool as a way to inform yourself about your own spiritual beliefs and how they line up with those who walk various other faith paths.

> We are all spirits, creatures of the divine, and all react to the things around us.
> The only way we can get through this life is through working together to create a better world.

YOU!

Our relationships with ourselves is the hardest part of our spiritual engagement. Now, while this may not feel spiritual to you, it is important to recognize that. There are many kinds of relationships we experience, including our relationship to our own bodies. We each have challenges we go through to keep our bodies well. Paying attention to our challenges helps open us up to new possibilities when interacting with other people. We must be selfish in this manner and take care of yourself first. You must be the most important thing to yourself. You matter! Tell yourself out loud; "I am a child of the divine existence and I matter!"

Take the time to think deeply about the questions below. While they may not show up in your life regularly, they define who you are and how you present yourself in the world. Take a breath before each question to center yourself on the topic you are approaching.

Who are you?

What makes you, you?

What things about yourself do you like?

What things about yourself do you not like?

What is your calling in life?

What steps are you currently taking to get there? (It is recommended to explore at least three)

What is causing you to struggle in life?

What, if you removed it from your life, would no longer allow you to be yourself?

GOALS

Having goals in life is what keeps us going. Without having goals, we would not be living our life to the fullest. When you have a goal, you enjoy the rewards and challenges that come with it. Always have big long term goals so you know where you want your life to be going. Along the way you will have many small goals that both direct you to your long-term goal, as well as little things that you think are fun and will add more fulfillment to your life. While I do not need to know how to make a quilted wall hanging for my long distant future, I am enjoying the joy and accomplishments that I am having along the way of learning this skill. Always wanting to move forward will add more pleasure to your life.

Setting goals is challenging. Working towards our goals is even harder. Refer back to the chapter on behavior change for more support in making and reaching your goals.

What do you want your life to look like?

What do you need to do to have this life you want?

What encourages you to reach for this life?

What are you called to do in life?

What empowers you to reach for your goals?

How can you include more of this in your life?

CARING FOR YOURSELF

What do you do to care for yourself? (It is recommended to explore three)

Do you care for yourself above all others?

What do you do for yourself to feel good?

What do you do for yourself to feel loved?

What do you do for yourself to relax?

What do you do that does not serve you? (It is recommended to explore three)

What do you include in your life that you do not enjoy?

What is missing from your life that would better it? (It is recommended to explore three)

ENCOURAGEMENT

Why do you live the life you currently do?

What can you do to be the best you?

What would enable you to have the life you want?

What do you do for yourself to encourage yourself?

What do you do for yourself to congratulate yourself?

CONTROL OF THE SELF

For some this is extremely challenging. All over the world there are people of all genders, races, and religions, that feel they are locked into boundaries that they did not define for themselves. Understanding your place in the world can help you to feel more in control, and help guide you to how you can function best within the constraints we are all limited by. Understand that there are very few individuals that have complete control over their own lives in this world. We can all start to bring it back into our control so that we are able to support the world and ourselves in the way we are meant to.

Do you feel in control of your own life?

Where in your life do you have the most control?

Where in your life are you lacking control?

Do you make decisions on how your life will unfold?

What choices put you in control of your actions and life? (It is recommended to explore three)

LABELING

While applying labels to yourself may not seem like a large thing, for some it is. Labels can cause us pain but they can also bring joy. Knowing how you interact with your own labels can be important to understand how you interact with the world and how you accept yourself for who you are. You are given the self-control, in this space in this time, to label yourself as you feel is your choosing. Empower yourself to become who you are in an opening up of possibilities. Try to not limit yourself but rather become larger than you are to encourage you to grow and reach towards your goals. You are not just a cashier. You are the person that gets to bring joy to each individual as they come to get what they need for the day, especially if it is a bad day. You are not just a person of color in the U.S.A. You are a strong person who, every day, overcomes silent adversity. You are not just an atheist. You are a person who exists in this world solely on their own merits.

What labels do you apply to yourself?

What of these labels encourages you to be larger than yourself?

What of these labels make you feel smaller than yourself?

Can you change the labels you apply to yourself to grow as a person?

PERSONAL SPIRITUALITY

As we start to get into more spiritually related things, understand this section is still about you, and not yet on your relationship with divine or spirit. We all have our own set of beliefs on how we exist, what we believe is important, and on how we act in this world. This is your own theory of how the world works. What do you really think rather than what you are told about the world?

What are your core beliefs on life? (It is recommended to explore three)

What are the most important ideas that guide how you live your life? (It is recommended to explore three)

How do you want to appear in the world?

What do you do to appear this way?

What do you do that is contrary to how you want to appear in the world?

Do you experience yourself as divine?

Are you worthy of receiving help, blessings, and support?

Does meditation and self-reflection have a place in your life?

What does a spiritual practice mean to you?

*What do **you** want to get out of having a spiritual practice?*

PERSONAL VALUES

What set of values do you adhere to in your life? (It is recommended to explore three)

Are these values you set, or were they set by others?

What happens to you when you cannot adhere to these values?

What rewards do you receive when you do adhere to these values?

THE BEGINNING AND THE END

When it comes to our personal beliefs on the world, much of our path is guided by how we believe we came into existence, and how we believe we will leave this existence. Here is a space to explore your ideas on these subjects, which may or may not follow any religious beliefs you understand. What are your personal ideas on these subjects? This can be the single most challenging thing we think about in our whole lives. Stop and really think. When you come closer to the end of your life, it will become more important for you to accept what you believe to be true about leaving this world. Take some time to begin this work now.

How do you believe you, as an individual, came to exist?

What are your thoughts on the creation of this existence and how we got to be here today?

What are your views on how you should live in the world?

What are your beliefs around death and after life?

How do you view the world in this existence?

ENVIRONMENT

As we saw from our introductory chapter, your personal environment can alter your impressions of the world greatly. Knowing how you interact with your space is important to understand so that you can make adjustments as needed. In this case, we are not yet interacting with others. For some, their spiritual path is a direct relationship with their environment. For others, colors and arrangements of furniture can greatly impact their own feelings about the world. How does your environment interact with you?

What in your personal environment serves you?

What do you need to add to your personal environment, or remove, so that it serves you better?

Where in life are you most yourself?

What about your environment makes you feel like yourself?

What can you do to alter your environment so it serves you better?

COMMUNICATION

While it is easy for most of us to communicate with others, it can be challenging to pause and think about situations with yourself. Sometimes we are scared to hear what we have to say, and other times we are angry at ourselves. It is important to recognize these moments, to accept them, and work to moving on and fixing or accepting the problems that led to these feelings towards yourself.

How do you communicate with yourself?

If you do not, would it serve you to check in on how you are doing?

How would you remind yourself to check in on how you are feeling in life?

How can you work towards accepting yourself for who you are?

CHAPTER 9: CONSCIOUS EATING, EXPLORING YOUR DIGESTION

Homework Assignment 7

Observe and record the following for a week.

- What food do you eat?
- How much of each food?
- What time do you eat?
- How do you feel physically after each time you eat food?
- How do you feel emotionally after each time you eat food?

Practice using the physical and emotional feeling words separately for your experience of your food. After each day, record any patterns you notice with how you 'feel' in relation to food.

FOOD EXPERIENCE

With this chapter focuses on being conscious of how food affects our body. Let us explore the different ways we can experience and interact with food.

Sight

The first experience we have with our food we will eat is seeing it. This can start us thinking about our food and what we are about to eat. This thinking starts the digestive process by increasing our production of saliva. We get other information from seeing our food as well. We can use our knowledge of food to know what we are eating, as well as what kinds of chemicals are in our foods such as protein, fats, or carbohydrates. As we discussed in the wellness input chapter, this information is useful to us for different functions of our bodies. Generally, this is the only way we have of distinguishing the different kinds of foods we are eating, and then we can decide if we are eating what we need. This is where you make a choice, when you can see and smell the food, to decide if you are going to eat it or not.

What are words you use to describe your food when you first see it?

Smell

Sometimes we can smell our food before we see it. This also helps promote the start of the digestive process. When we smell foods we are actually detecting small food particles in our nose. The signals of liking the smell or not, along with an idea on what the smell is, is sent to our brain to interpret it. There is a great theory that says that when something smells good to you, there are some molecules in there that your brain is detecting that it needs. This is particularly true of spices and is a great way to practice adding herbs and spices to your cooking. If it smells good it is probably something your body needs.

Smell is sometimes the first place we have physical reactions to our food. The same molecules we are interacting with in our nose, can prompt allergic responses in sensitive individuals. If something does not smell good to you, makes you sneeze or clear your throat, it is a message to you to pay attention. Some foods, like black pepper, will make most people sneeze because of the physical sensation of the molecules on the mucus membranes. Unless you know you are allergic to something, just pay attention to your reaction as you further process your experience with the food.

What are words you use to describe your food when you first smell it?

Are there any foods that elicit a response from you, positive or negative, from their smell?

Taste

We all experience our food through our mouth and for most of us, this is also the last place we think about our food experience during digestion. In Ayruvedic Medicine there are six different flavors we experience: sweet, salty, sour, bitter, astringent, and pungent. Each food is made up of a combination of these flavors, and we need a little bit of each of these in our diets. Most people like the sweet, salty, and sometimes the sour tastes on their own; but they need to be balanced with the bitter, astringent, and pungent tastes.

What tastes do you enjoy?

What foods do you eat that contain these tastes?

What foods could you eat to get the other tastes into your meal plan?

So what can each of these tastes tell us about the food we are eating and what our bodies need/want from our food? Some of these answers are easy. Sugar and sweet tastes are all of our carbohydrates that we need for our energy source. Salt, and salty foods, offer us the micro molecules we need for catalysts in various processes in our bodies. Salty flavors are often given from many minerals and is a reason you see dogs sometimes licking the ground, they taste salty minerals that they are lacking. Salts also allow our body more lubrication as the salts support our fluid balance, bringing in more water to our body with the salt.

89

The sour taste is usually vinegars and fermented foods. These fermented foods provide us with the microbiota that live in our digestive tract and through our entire body. Without these microbes, we would not be able to digest most of our foods and have appropriate pH balances for many of our enzymes to work. Arugula, and other greens like wood sorrel, also include the sour taste and similarly stimulate our digestion.

Bitter, pungent, and astringent are less easy to understand. The bitter flavor is often associated with detoxification support. Bitter molecules stimulate the gallbladder and liver secretions, allowing for a more efficient break down of fats and other compounds in the intestines. This liver support also helps to detoxify our bodies of everything from our own hormones, pharmaceuticals we take internally, and poisonous substances. The pungent flavor also stimulates our digestion, stimulating additional secretions, inducing gallbladder secretions to break down our food for better absorption. Astringent flavors tighten our tissues by pulling the water out of them. This can be important to maintain our fluid balance and offer enough fluid in our digestive tract to properly digest the food we eat.

Are there any effects of these tastes that you think you need more of?

Our sight and smell experience of food begins preparation in our mouths for food. Our taste receptors enhance this process, and start our stomachs releasing its digestive secretions. In our mouth we not only experience a variety of tastes, but we also experience a variety of textures. Texture does not really have any effects on our physiology, but it can affect our enjoyment of the food in our mouth.

What texture words do you use for your experience of food?

What is your experience of different food textures in your mouth?

Swallowing

This is an interesting place to experience your food but for me it has special significance. This is where I react to one of my food allergies. I pay attention best I can to the smell, sight, and taste of my food but as soon as I swallow I know if this allergen is in my food and my throat starts to close. It is a local reaction, and happens when the food touches my throat. After it passes there I have no additional observable reaction.

With a single bite it is challenging to make observations on what is happening when your body is interacting with the food. Take a moment now and swallow your saliva. How does it feel? As we get older the muscle control over swallowing can become reduced and it becomes important to know if our swallowing action is causing problems. It is also an area that we can detect food or allergens that end up in our lungs that shows up through coughing and respiratory difficulty.

What common sensations do you experience in your throat?

What do you notice when you swallow food? Water?

Do you notice anything as your food and water travel to your stomach?

Stomach

We experience very little of our food in our stomachs. Most often we are experiencing things in our intestines. Heart burn, acid reflux, and some gas can occur in response to food in the stomach. This is where our food is broken down with various acids and enzymes. Many things can alter the acids and enzyme activity, but this is not our focus now, our focus is observation.

How do you know when your food is in your stomach, not your esophagus or your intestines?

What feelings do you experience when food is in your stomach?

How do you explain these feelings from your knowledge of your body and food?

Generally, food sensitivities do not show up in the stomach, because no absorption is occurring, so the body does not have any food particles to react to. The only abnormal symptoms that one experiences in the stomach, is the body's method of starting the food break down process.

One of the most common of these is acid reflux, the over production of the liquids that break down our food. If this is a challenge you experience, when you are experimenting with food choices pay attention to what foods cause this symptom. Do you want to make the choice to eat them, and have the reflux, or do you want to make the choice to not have acid reflux symptoms?

Intestines

Many problems begin when food hits the intestines. Here we can actually feel lots of interactions with our food, when you know how to listen to your body.

What feelings do you experience when your food is in your intestines as an internal experience?

What feelings do you experience around your intestines as an external experience? (What does your abdomen feel like to touch?)

The intestines are where food starts to be absorbed, where our gut bacteria continue to break down food to be absorbed, and where bile from our gallbladder enters our digestive tract to break down fats so they can be absorbed. To summarize, it is where the remaining digestion and breakdown of food happens and where we start to absorb nutrients.

In our intestines, there is a whole other world of bacteria, microbes, that break down our food, or digest it for us, so we can absorb it more effectively. There are good and bad bacteria that live in our digestive tract. When there is a larger number of bad bacteria in the digestive tract they can both release irritating molecules, rather than good nutrients, and cause local inflammation and irritation to your intestinal lining.

If you are trying to improve the number of good bacteria in your intestines there are two ways to do it. You can choose to use prebiotics, the food that feeds the good bacteria, or probiotics. Probiotics are very common these days and are the actual bacteria that you need to have in high numbers in your digestive system. When you ingest probiotics daily, they outcompete the bad bacteria, taking over your intestines. Even if you take probiotics, it is a good idea to eat prebiotics to feed them so they do not get weak and let the bad bacteria take over again. Most fibrous plants act as prebiotics, and this is one of the many reasons to eat your vegetables.

After the food is digested by our bodies and our intestinal microbes, the food needs to be absorbed. Absorbing our food is when we have the most interaction with our food, as it finally enters our body. The particles we absorb all go to the liver, where they are transformed into usable sugars, fats, and protein particles to be transported through the body for use. When there is inflammation in the intestines, larger particles of food, those that should not be absorbed into the body, do get absorbed. These particles can be what cause allergic reactions and sensitivities to foods. This is often referred to as leaky gut syndrome, when we react to food that 'leaks' into our bodies when our intestines are inflamed, but food sensitivities can happen to anyone at any time in response to any food.

Other challenges that can occur here are the lack of ability to absorb nutrients. This can come if you have 'tanned' your intestinal lining by drinking fluids with lots of tannins. Tannins are molecules common in coffee and tea that make it dark colored and literally 'tan' proteins in the body, binding them together and preventing them from working, much like tanning a cowhide. Reducing coffee and tea intake can help this, as your body is constantly making new lining to your intestines. Other intestinal issues can arise from an inability to break down fats. Similar things can happen with other kinds of molecules and if your gallbladder is not supplying enough bile which aids in the breakdown of fats and other molecules.

However, the poor breakdown of food is hard to experience in the intestines. What we can often can feel is large amounts of inflammation. After you eat a meal many people feel 'stuffed.' This pressure is from a variety of different sources, including the obvious gas, but it can also be a result of an immune reaction. This reaction can be due to any number of irritating molecules being inappropriately absorbed into the body. You should never feel 'stuffed' after you eat. Take it as a sign that your food may be fighting back.

Do you ever experience actually looking heavier after eating? Looking and feeling like you ate so much that you could actually see that you gained weight from the meal? This is commonly called getting a 'wheat belly' and often comes in response to either wheat or dairy. It is an inflammatory response in the body with a collection of gasses fermented by your natural gut bacteria. Using clear feeling words, not emotions, to target what is going on, is important to choose what you are putting into your body, so you are able to determine if you are experiencing symptoms like this or if it is a much more serious problem like inflammatory bowel syndrome (IBS).

Do you ever notice changes in your body's physiology after eating?

Have you noticed any connections to certain foods that cause symptoms in your intestines?

What choices could you start to make regarding what you are eating to feel better?

Bowels

When it comes to our large intestines, our bowels or our colon, the most common symptom we experience is constipation. This can tell us a lot. What goes on in the bowels? When the remaining food particles come into the colon, they have been broken down as much as they are going to. The bowels are where we absorb the remaining food we will absorb as well as fluids, used to digest our food. It is very easy to see and smell what is going on in the bowels by what comes out. Before that happens, we've got to get the material out. Problems can come at this time if there is not enough fiber in the diet, or if you are dehydrated. When there is not enough fluid in the body, more fluid will be pulled out of the colon into the body, reducing the moisture in the digesta. Moisture hydrates the fiber allowing it to move through the colon faster. An additional reason why it is important to get the digesta to move is that the longer that it is in the colon, the more the bacteria in the digesta can ferment the material. This fermentation can cause gas and pressure in the lower abdomen.

How are your bowel movements? Frequency and ease?

What feelings do you experience in relation to the digesta in your bowels?

How does your body react to the feeling of an oncoming bowel movement?

What feeling words do you use to describe your bowel movements?

Sight and Smell (again)

As an herbalist, we often talk to our clients about their stool. We all love the Bristol stool chart which offers a wide variety of possibilities of visual descriptors of stool.

Bristol Stool Chart	
	Type 1: Separate hard lumps, similar to nuts. Hard to pass.
	Type 2: Sausage-shaped, but lumpy.
	Type 3: Sausage-shaped, but with cracks on the surface.
	Type 4: Sauage or snake-like, smooth and soft.
	Type 5: Soft blobs with clear-cut edges. Easy to pass.
	Type 6: Fluffy pieces with ragged edges, mushy.
	Type 7: Watery, no solid pieces. Entirely liquid.

What descriptors do you use to describe what your bowel movements look like?

Seeing and smelling our bowel movements can tell us a lot about what happened inside of our bodies to the food we ate. When you see food pieces usually it means you did not chew it properly for chemical break down to occur in the stomach. When you have different colored stool it can be from different foods you ate. If it is on the yellow end of the spectrum it can be because excess bile is released and not reabsorbed. If your stool floats it can be either a sign of reduced fat breakdown or of plenty of fiber in the diet. You will need to pay attention to what you are eating to know which of these is what is happening. Each descriptor can refer to things we want or don't want, so that is why it is important to pay attention to food in the rest of your body as well as knowing what you have put into your body. Many prescription medications can alter bowel movements, with most causing constipation, such as diuretic drugs.

You are what you don't poop.

This is a much better saying than 'you are what you eat.' The food that comes out in our stool is what we did not absorb in our intestines. Sometimes this can lead us to thinking about other challenges that may be going on in other places of our digestive track. One way to know a bit more about your digestion is to track the time it takes food to go through your digestive system. Beets can be used to track your food transit time, the time it takes you to eat to excrete. Pay attention to when you eat them and how many hours/days it takes for you to see purple in your bowel movements.

What can you tell about your digestion from your stool?

Urine

While what comes out in our stool was what was not absorbed into our body, everything that comes out in our urine was at some point absorbed into our body, transformed into something else, or used for something, before being excreted from our body. Two foods that many people have experienced through their urine are asparagus and beets. Some people will process the asparagus scent components, after they were absorbed, and they will not smell as they come out in the urine. Others do not process the scent components and will urinate out the scent. A separate gene allows you to smell the components so you may not know if you process it or not.

Our urine is the best way to also check our own hydration levels. Our urine should be clear to pale yellow if we are properly hydrated. A dark yellow indicates you should have more water in your system. Smells can also be an indicator of an imbalance in your body. If you notice an abnormal smell to your urine, seek a medical doctor.

What colors have you observed in your urine?

Have you noticed any smells from your urine?

On an average day, what does your urine smell and look like?

CHAPTER 10: MOVEMENT PRACTICE STAGE 2

Homework Assignment 8

For two weeks, do a full set of sun salutations twice minimally a day. They can be done at the same time. Record how your muscles feel before and after this practice each day.

I walk for 30 minutes a day, and I have been regularly standing for long periods of time.

If you are already able to stand and walk around with no problem for 30 minutes a day, you can start to add in more cardio activities and strengthening exercises as well. If you are not there yet you can skip this chapter and come back when you are. Start slow when starting to add cardio, stretching, and strengthening activities. Start where you feel comfortable, with movements that sound interesting to you.

When you start to increase your cardio movements, there are many possibilities of what you can do. Slowly increase your movement by regularly checking your heart rate to see where you are compared to your resting heart rate. At first, look to add in an additional 5 minutes a day of moderate intensity exercise. For most, when starting, this can be taking stairs slowly to not raise your heart rate too much, a light jog, or doing a higher energy dance to your favorite five-minute song each day.

Each week, replace an additional five minutes a day of your 30 minutes of walking exercise with moderate exercise. This means that week one, instead of doing thirty minutes of walking you will do twenty-five and five minutes of a more moderate exercise like jogging, dancing, or swimming. The next week, each day you will do ten minutes of moderate exercise and twenty minutes of walking. After a month and a half of this progression, you will then be reaching the goal as recommended by the AHA and ACSM. Congratulations!

POSTURE

Now that you have been walking for a little while you are probably starting to become more aware of your body and your posture. Having correct posture, and focusing on maintaining it, can benefit a variety of other health concerns including aiding in digestion and reducing pain. It is hard to learn correct posture, and it can be painful when you first start sitting and standing with a more appropriate posture, but it will only support the movement practices you are already adding in and get easier as you go.

Let's start looking at our posture by standing up. When you are just standing in line somewhere or cooking, any time when you are just standing still, take a moment to check in with how you are standing and shift so you are in a healthier posture. When checking on your posture, start with paying attention to your feet. Are your toes pointing forward and at a relaxed position apart from each other? Is your weight balanced between both legs? Move up your body. Are your knees facing forward and are they pointing over your toes?

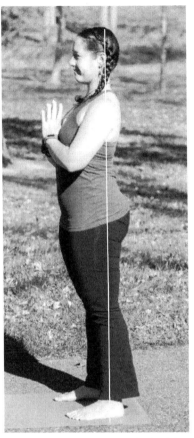

When you get to paying attention to your hips you may find you have a hard time knowing where your hips are positioned. Try rocking your hips side to side and forward and back. Don't tip your bowl, your hip girdle, too far to the front or the back. Individuals who are overweight tend to tip their hips forward. Individuals who are underweight tend to tip their hips backwards, sticking the hip bones forward. Try to find a place in between to hold while you are stationary. If you are not used to holding your hips in a good position, you may notice back pain when you shift your hips. This is normal and will go away as your muscles holding your hips in place get stronger.

Paying attention to your waist, engage your abdominal muscles and think of lifting your rib cage upwards so it is not resting and putting weight onto your spine. Continue to breathe when practicing this action as it can be challenging. Be sure to not allow any twists or bends in your waist. You can ensure this by checking that your shoulders are over your hips.

Relax your shoulders down, pulling the back of your shoulder blades towards each other in your back. This is another hard one for most of us. For individuals with larger chests, this will be extremely difficult to maintain for long periods of time. We get so used to hunching our backs forwards to relieve some of the weight, but pulling the shoulders back relieves our backs of the pain from the extra weight. Strengthening these muscles over time will reduce back pain associated with larger chest size.

In the following image, you are able to see the pulling together of the shoulder blades. While it is not an aim to be able to see your shoulder blades, this image is good to keep in the back of your mind to remember to bring your shoulders back as you present yourself to the world. This posture often will bring more confidence to you through your day.

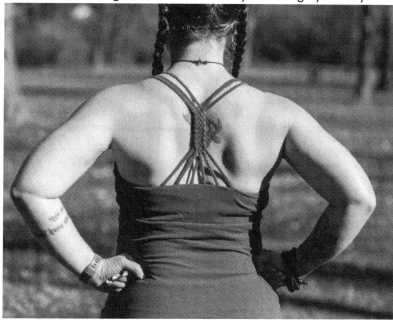

The last piece to check in with is your neck. The United States is just full of people with neck problems from hunching over a computer all day. When you think about your neck you want to focus on elongating it in the back and pushing your chin back slightly farther than you would normally hold your head. Again, this may be painful for a while, when practicing, until you learn to engage the correct muscles and strengthen them to hold your head properly.

It is very similar when you are sitting down to keep good posture. The waist and above should be just about the same. Even as I type now I am practicing this posture. The key for sitting however is having the right chair to promote positive posture. Most office chairs do not allow this. The best kind of chair to have is a solid wooden one that has a level seat, not one that is slanted backwards. Put your bottom on the middle front of the chair, feet both flat on the ground with knees and toes pointing forwards. You want your chair height to be about the same height as the length of your lower leg so when you sit you form a 90° angle at your knee. Keep practicing these posture techniques, and over time it will get easier and you will feel more comfortable in your body through the day.

Stretching and Strengthening

While the AHA and ACSM recommendations specifically refer to heart rate and time expenditure for exercise, they do not give additional

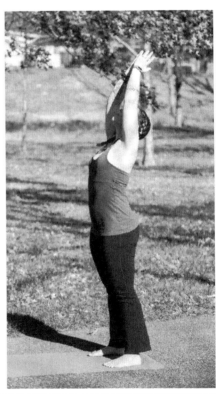

recommendations for stretching and strengthening practices. While it does not cover all muscular areas of the body, one of the best beginner practices, that includes both strengthening and stretching the larger muscles of the body, is doing a sun salutation.

A sun salutation is a combination of movements unique to yoga. If any of the movements here may challenge you, feel free to use a chair for support next to you, blocks under your hands for extra support, and be sure that the area around you is cleared so you are not at risk of hurting yourself from knocking into things.

Begin a sun salutation by standing with your feet about 6

inches apart (the length of a brick) with toes pointing forward. Relax your arms to your side and stand up tall. Be sure to lift your head. Be proud that you are doing something to serve yourself. Bring your arms up to your chest and push your palms together, pointing your elbows to the side, not back. Keeping your hands together bring your hands up to the celling and align your arms to your ears on the side of your head, not in front. You should feel a slight stretch backwards with your arms next to your ears. Feel free to very slightly bend backwards if you feel comfortable. Pause here for a moment and breathe.

Stand back up straight, release your hands from each other and turning your palms away from each other lower your arms to the sides. Continue bringing your arms downwards from this position, bending at the waist. Relax your body in a downward fold position, allowing your arms to relax towards the ground. Do not feel that you need to be touching the ground. The importance in this posture is relaxing your body into the weight of the earth. Do not forget to also relax your head. Pause here for a moment and breathe.

Bending your knees, place your hands on the ground (or on blocks) for stability. Step so that your right foot back as far as you can, still keeping your toes facing forward. If you are able to shift backwards and put your front heel down on the ground, do so. Keep your hands on the ground for balance and look up. Be proud, you have gotten this far in your

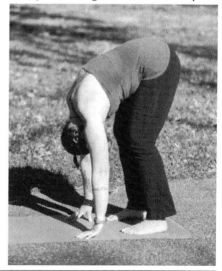

work. If you need to use a chair for balance you may want to also take a slightly smaller step backwards. In this lunge position, try to keep your toes and hips pointing forward. If you are not used to this position it may be very challenging at first. When you become more stable you can place your hands on your front knee. When you are in the position, pause for a moment and breathe.

Placing both hands back on the ground, swing your front leg back to meet your back leg. It is all

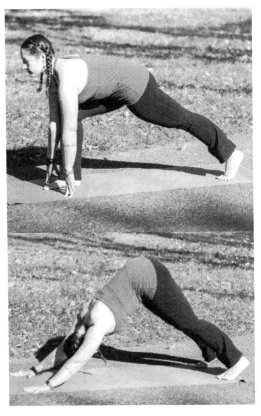

right if you need to put both legs down to then achieve them being behind you. Try to straighten both legs and arms, lifting your bottom up to the air and dropping your head down to the ground. This is the classic downward facing dog pose in yoga. It is not necessary that your heels are on the ground. If you are able to, remember the posture of your shoulders and be sure to rotate your shoulders down into your sockets and away from your ears. Pause here for a moment and breathe.

Now the next three are a bit more challenging. When you first begin doing a sun salutation you may choose to skip the next three and go right back into the other lunge.

From downward dog, keep your hands where they are and make sure your feet are again a brick distance apart. Lower your bottom towards the ground to create a straight line from your shoulders to your ankles, holding your waist in the air. Look up. This position is called the plank and helps to strengthen the arms. Remember your rotation of your shoulders and engage your stomach muscles to hold the position and breathe.

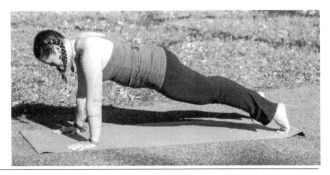

Relax your waist down to the ground and we will form the oddest step of the sun salutation called 8-points. You will place the 8 points on the ground and try to keep the rest of your body off the ground. Don't feel discouraged from this move. I think of this as the yoga version of wiggling. It is kind of silly, but it moves your body in a way it is not used to and helps you because it is different. The 8 points are, the toes on both feet, your two knees (so pop your heels up), your two shoulders and hands. This then means that your hips, elbows, and chin are ideally not on the ground, putting a gentle arch into your back.

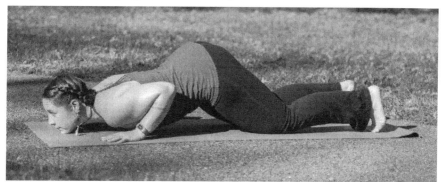

Continue to arch your back, resting your hips and feet down, lifting your head up. Think of bringing your chest forward. If you are able to do so, push into your hands and gently straighten your elbows. This is not necessary to get the stretch in your back. Pause here for a moment and breathe.

Lower your shoulders and head to the ground, turn your toes under, push into your hands again and pull your hips back up to the celling

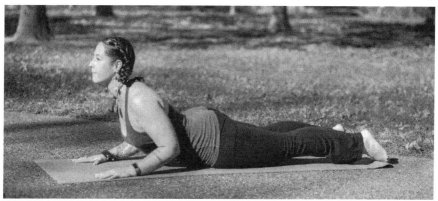

into downward dog again. Remember to relax your heels toward the ground but not onto the ground. Relax your head down and rotate your shoulders. Pause here for a moment and breathe.

Now transition back into a lunge with the other foot forward. If you brought your right foot back first, now bring your right foot forward. You can either swing your hips forward and pull your leg forward or go back to the floor and bring your right leg forward then raise from the ground. Remember to use a chair or blocks if you need for support. Try to straighten your back leg with your toes forward. If you have the stability you can raise your hands to your legs from the floor. Pause here for a moment and breathe.

Place your hands on the ground and pull your back leg forward to meet your front leg. Be sure to have your feet a brick distance apart. Straighten your legs up as much as possible, relaxing your arms and head towards the ground. Pause and breathe in this forward fold.

Extend your arms out to the sides, straighten your legs and stretch your back straight, raise your body upwards to stand. Feel free to use a chair for this if needed. When upright with your arms out, raise your arms over your head and press your palms together, arms at your ears. Allow for a gentle backwards bend and breathe.

Straighten your body up, and bring your arms back down, palms still together, in front of your chest. Breathe here for a minute and then begin again, this time initiating the lunges with the left foot rather than the right. Always do the progression twice through so you are able to initiate the movements with each side. This will encourage balance in your workout.

While this sequence can be challenging to a beginner, it contains a little bit of everything. There are many alterations you can make to this sequence to fit your needs. I am all for taking advantage of free technology. There are many videos online and free apps to help teach you how to do a sun salutation properly. Don't forget to do both sides. Repeat the movements a second time bringing a different foot forward for lunging each time.

I recommend starting with doing one cycle, or repetition, every other day, holding each position for 20-30 seconds, or as long as comfortable, until you start until you become familiar with the sequence.

Once you become familiar with the sequence, slowly increase the amount of time you hold positions for the strengthening and stretching benefits or move through the sequence more quickly, increasing your heart rate for a cardio work out. For the first few weeks that you do this kind of movement, do this sequence every other day before increasing your frequency and repetitions. This will give your body time to adjust and heal to the new movements. You may however increase the number of times you do the sequence slowly. Always go slow. You will be more successful long term if you work towards consistency at a slower pace.

At this point in your movement practices, if you want more, I recommend starting to take beginner classes in movement that interest you. Yoga is an excellent option, and many Yoga classes are not expensive, but it is not for everyone. The Sun Salutation is a good overall movement program to start adding more stretching and strengthening, making this Yoga practice good for beginners. Try some different activities until you find one you love and can stick with!

CHAPTER 11: SUCCESSFUL SLEEP PATTERNS

Homework Assignment 9

For two weeks, set an alarm to wake up at the same time each morning, even on days you have off. Record what time you go to bed and how you feel in the morning.

We spend one third of our lives sleeping. Or, we probably should spend about one third of our lives sleeping. We all know that sleep is something we struggle with. We will get to talking about finding what sleep methods work best for you, but in the meantime let's talk about why we need sleep and delve more into the benefits of sleep.

> The Division of Sleep Medicine at Harvard Medical School states: Sleep is a state that is characterized by changes in brain wave activity, breathing, heart rate, body temperature, and other physiological functions.

Sleep is a time when we are unconscious, and yet we are able to easily regain consciousness. Some of the time, while we sleep, our brains are just as active as when we are awake. It is interesting to note that the difference in brain waves shows up as more ordered waves, organized patterns, while asleep. When awake, we receive a lot of stimuli that alter our brain waves and create disorder. Sleep allows us to relax our mental processes and gives us order even without our awareness.

There are 5 stages we experience while we sleep. Though we do not often remember them, even when we are sleeping through the night we have brief moments of wakefulness. Usually these do not disrupt our sleep. As we start to fall asleep and are in our lightest stage of sleep we experience REM sleep. This rapid-eye-movement stage is where our dreams occur and when our brain is functioning similar to when we are awake. The next stage is known as N1. This first nonREM sleep stage is easy to wake from and is when we will still wake from body movement. The N2 stage is where we spend about half of our night sleeping. N3 is our most deep sleep stage. It is hard to wake someone in this stage but it can be done. When woken from this stage it can take **up to an hour for the body to recover completely**. In the N3 stage the breathing becomes regular, the pulse slows, and our core body temperature lowers.

While we sleep our blood pressure, and body temperature drop. The lowest pulse rate you experience when awake comes from lying down when you have just woken up. Before even sitting up, taking your pulse rate will determine what we call your basal pulse rate, your base line to use when exercising. Our temperature reduction is to conserve energy, an almost hibernation overnight. This hibernation and relaxation of all of our systems while we sleep also gives our heart a rest with the lower blood pressure and pulse rate.

While all of these processes slow down, others speed up. The most interesting is an increase in growth hormone while we sleep. This may contribute to our bodies repair mechanism while we sleep. Our digestion is increased as well as cell growth and tissue repair. This is essential to our body, and, as discussed in the conscious eating chapter, protein is what is needed for tissue repair so of course our digestion will need to be working while we are sleeping and repairing our body. We need to absorb the nutrients we need to repair our body as well as process these nutrients.

The benefits to sleep are obvious. Sleep allows us to recuperate, heal our bodies, strengthen our memory pathways, relax our cardiovascular system, and often process things that are more challenging, within our dreams. Truly, the reason that sleep makes us feel better immediately, is not from getting sleep but rather the act of not being awake. So let's look at how we normally experience sleep.

What time do you generally start to prepare for bed?

What is your general pre-sleep ritual?

What time do you turn off your lights and settle to sleep?

What is your experience from this time until you fall asleep, generally?

Do you wake at all, that you are aware, while you are sleeping? Does this disturb your sleeping?

What do you do to return to sleep if you are woken in the middle of the night?

Do you wake to go to the bathroom and have trouble returning to sleep?

What prompts you to wake up in the morning? At what time?

How does your body respond to waking up?

Does it take you time to adjust to being awake?

Homework Help

This week, work on waking up at the same time every day of the week, including weekends. Over time, waking up regularly will encourage your body to take over its rhythms of sleep. Encourage yourself to set an alarm and get up on the first ring. Avoid the temptation to snooze! Jump right out of bed. It will be jarring if you are not used to it. These weeks are also ideal to play with adjusting the temperature of the room you sleep in. Often, cooler spaces are more comfortable to sleep in, but we need to balance that so we do not get so cold we stay awake. And NO napping this week.

Afterwards, feel free to continue to experiment around sleep. Sleep really is key to most of our ability to function during the day, so having a sleep schedule that works for you is very important. Having good sleeping habits can encourage us to sleep well, but they still may not encourage an ideal sleep pattern every night. Even I have herbal and nutritional sleep aids next to my bed and, we will talk about some of them later in this book. For now, focus on sleep without supplements to support your body getting into its own rhythm.

WHY IS A SLEEP SCHEDULE IMPORTANT?

Our body naturally goes through cycles. We evolved with cycles of the yearly seasons, and a cycle of day and night daily. These cycles are set up around the light and dark cycles, and the rotation of the earth on its axis, altering the angle of the sun's rays hitting the earth. Within our bodies we also experience cycles such as, the menstrual cycle in women, as well as our sleep cycle. This sleep cycle is known as our circadian rhythm and is directly altered by the light we experience during our day.

As the sun sets and our bodies start to prepare for sleeping, the levels of melatonin in our bodies start to rise. This occurs when we are relaxing, preparing for bed, and have lower light levels. Our highest levels of melatonin usually occur between midnight and 2am. While we sleep, our body uses this melatonin to begin cortisol production. In the morning, cortisol helps our bodies to wake up and prepare for the day.

Cortisol is known to many as the stress hormone, as it gets higher when our bodies are stressed. It increases our heart rate, blood pressure, and our temperature, helping us to wake up in the morning. However, when we are more stressed this cortisol level can encourage us to stay awake. This is the primary reason that people who are stressed have a hard time falling asleep. Keep this cycle in mind as you look at some of the techniques to support your body's natural rhythms.

Two simple things that I do when my sleep schedule is a bit messed up is choosing to keep my blinds open on my windows in my bed room. This allows for natural light to wake me up in the morning. Going camping also has a similar effect with light. It is said that seven days of camping is enough to reset your natural body's sleep rhythm. I have experienced this first hand, and I think it is a valuable tool for supporting your sleep when you really need a kick to get in gear.

Now you are probably sitting there thinking, "I can do something else and still improve my sleep." Stop that thought right now. If you actually want to get better sleep, feel well rested, and improve your ability to function during the day, you need to stop messing around and fix your sleep schedule. If you think you can skip this, you need to seriously accept that there is no other real way to fix your sleep and sleep more effectively. NONE! So step up and take control of your life, and get to bed and wake up at the same time every day.

PREPARING FOR BED

It is important to have a good bed time routine, because several things can all contribute to how you experience going to sleep. The first, is how caffeine effects our sleep patterns. Many people use caffeine as a drug to keep them awake during the day, and to wake up in the morning. I believe caffeine is a great method of regulating your wake sleep cycle when it is taken in the morning, only in the morning, and in an amount that works for you. For most people, they need to stop having caffeine by about noon to prevent all effects from caffeine in the evening. Then there are others who can have a full cup of coffee and fall asleep five minutes later; this is unusual.

Experiment for yourself and try to not feel attached to your caffeine. Think of all of the rewards you will gain from having a good night sleep after not having caffeine. Shifting this habit can be difficult and stressful. Take your time. You can ease yourself down from caffeine, or just go cold turkey. Adjust your intake for what serves you best. Keep in mind, you will also be saving a significant amount of money over time if you buy coffee at a coffee shop. Even one cup a day will work out to about $140 in savings a month at a place like Starbucks.

How do you interact with caffeine through the day?

Is this serving your sleep and wake cycles?

What adjustments to your caffeine intake could support your sleep wake cycles?

Food can cause problems when eaten right before bed. Even though we digest food while we sleep, it is primarily being digested and absorbed in our intestines and not in our stomach. Consider stopping eating an hour or two prior to bed, at least, to reduce the digestion occurring in your stomach while you are lying down to sleep. It is interesting that even though reducing eating before bed is recommended, some foods can support us sleeping more effectively. For some people, a gluten sensitivity shows up as making one feel tired. This can serve you if it is your only symptom from eating gluten. (This may be one reason why marketing agencies have started promoting cereal before bed.) It all makes sense now!

Have you observed any food that alters your sleep?

Have you observed any food that alters your energy levels? Could this support your sleep cycle?

Lights are another thing we have complete control over when planning for bed. Our bodies evolved outdoors with the rhythms of the sun and moon. When we turn the lights down prior to bed it tells your bodies to start preparing and relaxing for bed. This is why candle lit dinners are more relaxing to us. By blocking windows if you are in a well-lit neighborhood you have more control over the lighting in your bedroom.

Light works the same way in the morning. I always recommend to keep window shades open when sleeping, if you can, to allow morning light to enter to help us slowly wake up with the sun rising. If this is not possible, there are alarm clocks and lamps that slowly increase the light in a room to promote waking up. If your sleep challenges are more in waking up this can be great support. It is also due to light that we often have challenges with our sleep when the seasons shift. We start to get different amounts of light each day. Regulating this indoors is something we can do now to keep our schedule normal.

It can also be a huge challenge to put down the electronics before going to bed. Just looking at a screen can reduce your ability to fall asleep. Take some time before bed without electronics. Set your alarm and then do something else for the last hour before you go to bed. Your phone will be there in the morning. Play around with this to see if it works for you. Generally, it is the light from the phone that is detrimental. Take some 'you time' before bed rather than playing games or watching videos.

Do you practice diming the lights in the evening or allowing light to enter your room in the morning as you wake?

Are you affected by light sources that enter your space as you sleep such as clocks, street lights, or digital screens?

What changes to the light in your space could you make to support your sleep cycle?

Being able to sleep with sound is something that is very individualized. Most of us are around sounds all day long. When we go to sleep and turn sounds off, it can be very relaxing for some while for others it can be more stressful. For myself I enjoy having sounds while I am relaxing and preparing for bed. Light affects me more. Reducing or changing sounds can promote different emotional responses, helping to prepare us for bed. For example, think of times when you listen to music you like to lift your mood. Music can also be used to calm us and prepare ourselves for bed. Other options include turning off the television, calming the kids down, reducing conversation, and allowing for more inward thoughts.

What sounds are relaxing do you? Stressful?

What kinds of sounds do you need, or don't need, while you are trying to sleep?

While all of these items are relaxing and calming, generally, we don't think of exercising as part of our bed time routine. A brief amount of exercise before bed can actually be a great way to center yourself, increase endorphins, and get blood out of your head and into your muscles for healing support while sleeping. Exercising can regulate your breathing and with the shift in blood you can even reduce thinking about a variety of worries. If you have trouble winding down, getting your excess energy out is one option through exercising. For most, this does not need to be much movement to get these simple effects before bed. For kids even ten jumping jacks will suffice. I have a little five-minute routine that I will sometimes do including traditional Pilates and Yoga moves.

Distractions to sleep are so common. Partners and pets sometimes will wake us, but we love them so we find ways to work with them. It is becoming more common for partners to sleep in separate beds, but this may not necessarily work for you. Larger beds can also help you sleep with less distractions as well, but having clear communication between you and your partner can be important to determine what you each need to receive the best sleep.

Pets can be more challenging because they like to cuddle, and we can't tell them no easily. Having a special blanket or bed on your bed can give your pet an area to sleep in that is special to them and close to you at the same time. If you suffer from allergies to your pet I do not recommend allowing them in the bedroom. This will only aggravate your allergies. It may take some time for your pet to get used to not being in your room, but in the long run you will be much happier this way.

With all of these techniques, the most important thing is consistency. Consistency in doing them and at the same time every night. Setting up a rhythm and pattern is the key to sleep health. This consistency includes consistency in waking up at the same time every day, and is why setting an alarm for weeks three to four supports a healthy sleep pattern. It is hard at first to set up these schedules, but once you get going you will not need an alarm and it will be just like riding a bike, you will just get it and keep going eventually. Practice can be hard, so keep working at it.

GUIDED MEDITATION

Continuing with our bed time preparation, other things that we can include in our relaxation prior to bed can include a meditation period using breathing techniques. Practicing breathing meditations in the early evening has helped me to fall asleep easier than practicing when I am trying to fall asleep. Other relaxing guided meditations can serve you in addition to breathing practices. In yoga, the shavasana pose, or the dead man's pose, is one of lying flat on the back and meditating in that pose without falling asleep. If you are new to meditating, falling asleep in this pose is very common.

There are many electronic applications that can be used to listen to while you are falling asleep if you can have sound in your space. These can include spoken meditations that will guide you through relaxing individual portions of your body in a systematic way. Others offer a variety of music and sounds that you can adjust to suit your relaxation and meditation needs. One new feature that more apps are offering are binaural beats. These beats that you add to your music are thought to directly influence brainwaves depending on the frequency. 10Hz is recommended for relaxation and 20Hz for concentration meditations. A lower wave length of 8Hz may be ideal for preparing the body to fall asleep, and similarly, it can support waking up as well. These binaural beats require headphones to work so playing them out loud on a phone or computer is not effective. There are however, isochronic tones that are thought to work very similarly and can be played through a phone or computer speaker.

STAYING ASLEEP

This is the hardest part to support and deal with, waking up in the middle of the night. Our natural sleep patterns often have us waking up briefly and falling back asleep without us ever knowing. Sometimes we don't fall back asleep and our bodies are ready to be active, or at least not asleep any longer. Many people end up taking drugs to prevent this from happening and that is one possible strategy. For others, being awake in the middle of the night has become habit for one reason or another. A few supportive habits can reduce this from happening.

When you wake up and cannot fall back asleep quickly it is best to just get up and do something. This can be anything from starting a load of laundry, doing a bit of exercise, reading, going to the bathroom, or even having a snack if you woke because of hunger or thirst. I do not recommend turning on screens - phone, television, or otherwise. Now, even I use my phone as a clock all night long, but I also know that if I look at it in those brief moments while I am awake I can become more alert. Even seeing the time on a lit-up clock can make me anxious as I try to sleep, reducing the effectiveness of my sleep. Pay attention to what techniques of falling back asleep have worked well for you in the past, and try to repeat them. This is one reason why journaling your experiences is so important to learning your best wellness practices.

If you do wake up and then fall back asleep after a time, be sure to still wake up at the same time you normally do. Keeping a rhythm is the key to sleep health, and even this reduction in sleep volume will support you because it will encourage your next night of sleeping to be more full.

WAKING UP

As I have said before, making and keeping a rhythm is the key to sleep health. Waking up at the same time every day, even on the weekends, can really support a healthy sleep pattern. Alarms can be really helpful for setting this up and maintaining a consistent pattern.

Setting up a wake-up schedule can be just as hard as setting up a sleep schedule. When your body wakes up to an alarm, and it was in the middle of a REM cycle it can take up to an hour to feel awake. This is why we so often hit snooze on our alarms. Tracking how long you sleep each night, and how you feel when you wake up after different lengths of sleep will help you target how long your REM cycles are, and when you should wake up. 3-5 REM cycles in 8 hours is common but they can also be at different lengths.

When you have to wake up in a REM cycle, do not rely on caffeine every day to get you to wake up faster in that first hour. Excessive caffeine is something that really cripples our society as a whole and prevents us from having a healthy sleep cycle. Everyone is capable of finding a balance between going to sleep and waking up, the time slept, and their daily schedule. It will be hard but keep at it. Having caffeine every so often, on those nights that you woke up for a few hours in the middle of the night, or the morning of a big presentation after staying up late to finish the preparation, it is alright. Remember it is a choice that could then upset your sleep cycle if it is secure without caffeine.

For those of you who 'can't survive without caffeine' there is another thing to consider. Caffeine, though it is a natural substance that appears in plants we grow, it is still a drug and can be an addictive substance. Caffeine withdrawal is not uncommon when people choose to reduce their amount of caffeine. If you are not having trouble sleeping do not worry about it so much. If you are having trouble sleeping, and you have caffeine often, it is the first place to start looking at to support your sleep schedule.

Napping in the day can be a tool to support your mood, energy, and healing process through allowing your body extra rest in the middle of the day. This is definitely an area where experimenting and finding what works best for you is super important. A nap at the wrong time for the wrong length of time, can mess up your sleep schedule for days. To help with this, when you do choose to nap, make sure you set an alarm. The worst thing to happen could be to take a nap while on your lunch break and not get back to work. Experiment with naps when you are not at work to find the length of nap that works best to leave you feeling refreshed. If your nap is too short, or too long, it can leave you feeling even groggier afterwards. This is due to which portion of your sleep cycle you wake from. Remember, waking in some phases of your sleep cycle can leave you feeling worse for up to an hour after waking.

CHAPTER 12: YOUR RELATIONSHIP TO OTHERS

We all have our limits, and it is important to know yours. Some of the following questions may be uncomfortable to consider, but it is important to know yourself when it comes to these challenges. We are often limited by our own fears in our relationships to others. Learning more about yourself, and how you interact with others, will help remedy this. Also, learning what you need to receive from others, and yourself, to have fruitful interactions with others, will support you on a path to happiness in this life.

Which of your interactions with others are important to you?

What are your three main goals of interactions with others?

SUPPORT

Who supports you?

Who do you support in response?

What do you do to support others without being asked to do so?

HOW TO TREAT OTHERS

What are your views on how you should treat others?

Do you actively treat others this way?

Do you encourage others to treat you this way as well?

What do you do to include others in your life?

What do you do that excludes others from your life?

What would cause you to verbally, physically, or mentally harm someone?

What do you do to reduce yourself harming others?

LANGUAGE AND COMMUNICATION

Many of the communities I am involved with view language as a very important piece of our interactions with other people. The strongest issue I come across is the use of pronouns to define the genders of individuals. While I am no expert in this area, what I have learned through this communication is that it is best to be open to new possibilities of how to interact with others. I always approach situations as a beginner, in a place of unknowing, so that I may learn from another what their view is, so I can adjust my language and speech in a way that will reduce any upset from occurring. This is great in many cases where gender is a spectrum, in cases where race, religion, or spirituality are being discussed, as well as in business meetings where you need to make sure everyone is understanding the same words you are using. Understanding, being open to different interpretations, is what makes communication possible between different people.

*What words do you use that **include** other people and possibilities?*

What words do you use that exclude other people and other possibilities?

What labels do you apply to others that encourage them to be larger than they are in your eyes?

What labels do you apply to others that reduce them in your eyes?

How can you change the labels you apply to others to shift your relationship with them?

What verbal tools do you use to communicate with others? For example, "I don't understand; can you elaborate?"

*What challenges **you** when communicating with others?*

What gets in the way of having clear communication with others?

Communicating with others and working together is the only way we will make in through this life in a way that feels positive. When you are open to new possibilities in conversations with others, you accept them for who they are and their ideas. You do not have to believe their ideas.

Accepting other ideas of others, as being equal to your own, will create a stronger platform for discussion and more effective outcomes. Thank people when they are open to working with you this way. Not just through verbal thanks, but also by being open to working with them in the same way. If they are not able to be open, open up to them and show them how efficient it can be to be open to other possibilities.

The more you are open, the more other people will be open to you in response. It is a cycle, like most things, where we can only spread positive interactions through releasing fear and anger and creating clear communication. When you struggle in this area, go back and think on what is challenging you in having clear communication. We cannot change others; we can only change ourselves and only when we make the conscious choice to do so.

COMMUNITY VALUES

Do you consider yourself part of a larger community? What defines this community?

What is the set of values that unite this community? (It is recommended to thinking of at least 3 unifying values.)

Which of your personal values line up with this community?

Which of your personal values do not line up with this community?

How do you respond to the values that do not line up?

OTHER COMMUNITIES

Are there communities of people with whom you do not agree with their beliefs, doctrines, or actions? Why?

What do you do that excludes them from your life?

What do you do that includes these people in your life?

What can you/do you do to accept these people for who they are?

What can you/do you do to work with these people to find common ground?

What are your thoughts on how others should live their lives?

As discussed before, it can be really challenging to work with people that have different beliefs and values than ourselves. When I was looking for guidance in relation to this, I looked out my window and saw two pairs of black birds fly by. The four birds were not flying alone, nor were they flying all together, they were flying as two pairs. Now while it is probably mating season, it made me think that as we go along our own path, we will find others that want to travel with us, and we will find others that do not want to travel with us, instead travel with others. We are all still worth wile regardless of the path we are following, and we must recognize this. There will be times when we are all in the same place and need to work together for common goals, and then separate to go on our own again. We need to be open minded and open to new possibilities. Reducing judgment and finding common ground is one way to do this.

EXPECTATIONS

Commonly, when we end up judging others, it is because we have certain expectations on how people should or should not act or experience the world. I would love to have the expectation that everyone with this book reads the whole thing, but I am not expecting that to happen. While reducing and lowering expectations can be one way to deal with any upset that may come along, I think it is more important to have clear communication with others to determine what appropriate expectations are.

Expectations may change over time, and being open to communication will help keep everyone from having more than their share of upset over the situation. It can be hard to do this with people you do not know. Not everyone is going to be able to meet your expectations of them, no matter what these expectations might be. I may expect someone to arrive on time to an event, but being open to the possibility that that may not happen will reduce my own upset. You do not have control over another being. Having expectations suggests that you do have control over their actions.

Do you expect more from others than they are able to offer you?

How could you work with individuals to best support each other?

Look back at what you your thoughts on how others should live your lives were. Can you reasonably expect others to do this?

While it would be nice to have all of our expectations filled, it is not something that is helpful for us to expect of them. Every individual is in control of themselves and we cannot change what they choose to do, regardless of how clear we make our expectations to them. When it comes to life choices, even if we think everyone should do a certain thing, we cannot expect it from everyone. This not only harms others by expecting change, but is also harms ourselves through lowering out trust and confidence in others. It is hard to release expectations of others, and I myself am constantly working on it. It is very rewarding when you are able to accept others for who they are and their own abilities.

CONTROL AND PERMISSION

Sometimes we have to take control away from another individual to protect them. An easy example of this is taking away car keys from someone who has had too much to drink. There are, however, other times where it is not appropriate to take away someone's control over their life. It can be challenging because different individuals need control in different areas of their life. When in doubt, always ask permission rather than taking something from someone. You never know how it will affect them. A simple thing, such as a hug, can cause damage if done at the wrong time in the wrong place. Verbal permission is always best, however we may not always be able to clarify to others what our needs are in a moment.

You are not in control of the actions of others. What can you do to reduce your upset in response to the actions of others?

How do you react to others when they attempt to take away your own control?

Have you been in a situation when you have taken control over another person? Did this person give you permission to do so?

What can you do to work with an individual trying to take away your control away when you did not give them permission?

INTERACTIONS WITH NON-HUMANS

Generally, when we think of our interactions with others we are thinking about humans. It is important to most of our value systems that we also think about how we interact with plants, animals, and the earth itself. While for some this may also be an interaction with divine, interacting with other humans can also be an interaction with the divine, depending on your definition. It is important to recognize that all interactions are important in one way or another. and caring for your pets or for your chickens can be just as important as caring for an apple tree or your neighbor. All of these interactions are important and acknowledging this and treating all beings with respect, will not only help you care for the others but will also fill you with pride and accomplishment. This should not be limited to the beings you come into contact with. Just like with treating others the way you want to be treated, you should also consider treating the earth and communities with this same respect and openness.

Do you interact with plants and animals with the same respect you do with other humans? Why or why not?

What about the earth? Do you treat and care for it with the same respect?

Do you encourage others to treat animals, plants, and the earth with the values you have?

What can you do to improve your interactions with animals, plants, and the earth?

CHAPTER 13: MAKING GOOD FOOD CHOICES

Homework Assignment 10

Go back and review all of your food related journal entries. Look through them and see if any patterns emerge of foods that are supporting you or ones that are not supporting you. Choose one food to eat more of and one to not eat at all. Continue with this choice for two weeks and record how you feel after meals in response to your change in meal plan.

This assignment may be one that you need to repeat over and over again until you find that you are having pleasant experiences after all meals.

If you are not used to listening to your body it can be very challenging to allow yourself to open up. We are always trying to reduce our emotional responses, and many of us have symptoms that we hide so we do not have to deal with them. Think of the last time you were sick. Were you still coughing or blowing your nose weeks after you were sick, but not taking any medicine to help you get better? We try to minimalize the importance of our symptoms so we can move on with our lives. This makes it hard to pay attention to them when we need to.

The most common method of checking on different parts of your body is through meditation, but a full meditation session, of ten or more minutes is not necessary every time you need to think clearly about how your body is feeling.

Practicing meditation consistently can make it easier to check in with the rest of your body. Additional discussion on meditation techniques can be found in the appendixes. For the time being, take a moment to breathe and try to relieve yourself of all of the thoughts in your head. From there, to practice checking in on the different parts of your body, start at your feet and pay attention to them for a few moments. Slowly move up the body, focusing on each region of the body as you go. Let your body tell you what it needs to. If you commonly have pain you ignore, this may be an uncomfortable experience. I tend to start to get back aches when I review my entire body like this. Practice this daily to be able to focus on individual areas when you need to rather than your entire body.

Another excellent method of checking in is through journaling and free writing, if you are more a visual rather than a kinesthetic learner. Have a small notebook or journal to carry around with you during your explorations. Use it to record what you are eating and your experiences with food. To practice, write what comes to you about how you are feeling. Over time you can start to focus on writing about the physical feeling words rather than emotional words we often write about. Remember, emotions are important too and should be used when making choices after we are clear in what we are feeling physically.

For auditory learners, a great method is to talk it out alone or with a partner. You can talk to your body parts and reply as if you are just that piece alone to focus on that area. Talking out possibilities so you can hear different experiences about a certain region can be supportive in presenting ideas to answer yes or no to.

What method of checking in is working well for you?

What parts of your body are you noticing feelings in?

Remember to check in

Once you have started to know how to check in and know where to listen to your body, it becomes a challenge to remember to check in.

How could you remind yourself to check in on your body?

You can find something you do before eating and make a mental note that every time you do it that you will also check in with your body. Some of the things we often do before eating that can remind you to check in are pouring a glass of water, washing your hands, taking out dishes, or turning off the car engine before going to a restaurant. While eating you can check in every so often to see if you are still feeling pleasant. If you are not, stop eating, drink water, walk around, and check back in with your body to see if it would serve you to continue. This is not always necessary, but in the beginning, as you are becoming aware of your interactions with food, it can serve to take your time with each eating of food.

Check back in again about two hours after eating to see how your body is processing the food you ate. About that time, it will be getting to your intestines and a reaction can occur. Generally, foods that irritate us often do not start to affect our physiology until they start to be absorbed in the intestines an hour or two later.

At this point, you have not probably changed much about what you eat, and that is fine. This chapter is not intended to have you change, but only to experiment with and see how your body reacts to different foods. There are many different food trends out there and some will work for you and some will not. It is important to discover what works best for your body. We are going to take a bit of time now to talk about some healthy eating habits you can explore to determine what works best for you.

One of the largest food related issues right now is the idea of food being organic and free of GMOs. Organic food means that it is grown without pesticides, for killing insects, and herbicides, for killing weeds and other plants. Clearly, eating organic food is going to be better for the environment, with less chemical killing of pests and plants that keep the ecosystem thriving. But does it really do anything better for your health?

Besides removing the pesticides and herbicides from your own diet, organic food has been found to be up to 70% higher in nutritional content. I was ecstatic when a study done by Rodale Institute in 2014 found this. If you are feeling that you are not getting enough nutrients out of your food, and you do not want to increase the calories, going organic is an excellent option.

Organic food can be expensive. Buying in bulk is one option for reducing the cost, and another is buying locally at a farmer's market or through a CSA, Community Supported Agriculture, directly from a farmer you know. When you are purchasing food from a farmer's market be sure to ask the farmer if the food is organic. Not all farmer's markets require all produce to be organic so be sure to check. Many other farmers grow their produce organically but do not pay for the certification.

If you cannot afford to transition completely to organic food, there is another option you can also consider. Each year a list is put out of the 'Dirty Dozen' and the 'Clean Fifteen.' The Dirty Dozen is a list of 12 plants that are considered to be highest in herbicide and pesticide residue. I recommend starting by purchasing these foods organic. On the other end, the Clean Fifteen are the lowest in herbicides and pesticides which make them better choices when you cannot eat organic. Applications for your phone are easily found that keep these lists updated and at your easy reach. Following the recommendations on these two lists can greatly help reduce your intake of potentially dangerous chemicals in your food.

GMO, or genetically modified organism, is a term that is very broad, and can include everything from selectively breeding cows for the best tasting meat, to the addition of new genetic material to a plant or animal, usually from another plant or animal, but sometimes one that is entirely made by scientists in a laboratory. There is a large amount of debate over whether or not GMOs are safe and healthy to eat. I recommend doing just what we have been doing. Eat and see how it feels and works in your body. Each GMO ingredient is different and will affect each of us differently. The chemically modified GMOs have not been tested for long term effects yet, so we do not really know potential effects, so it is best to experiment for yourself.

There is another concern regarding GMOs that you may or may not be aware of: their environmental impact. These new genes are grown in plants and animals, and then through breeding the genes change over time and spread through the entire population and system. We have no clue the long-term effects of introducing these new genes to a new system. It could do nothing, or it could cause great harm and cause disastrous damage to the plant's population, potentially wiping out the species if it is problematic enough.

When you choose to eat your foods, be sure to be investigating where it came from and how it was grown, so you can make the choice to eat it or not. As a consumer, you get to vote by what you buy. If you buy organic, the food industry will grow more organic foods that are healthier for our environments and for the people. It is expensive sometimes, but do what you can and over time, even the organic food will reduce in price as consumers show that they want more of it.

Another group of foods you may want to pay attention to are your simple and complex carbohydrates. A simple sugar/carbohydrate is what you think of when you think of as sugar. It is that sweetness that gives you a quick energy rush when you eat it. Complex sugars are more of your grains, beans, and vegetables. These carbohydrates take longer to break down in your digestion, offer higher amounts of nutrients and fiber, and generally sustain you for longer periods of time.

As you experiment with your food, if you notice that you are low in energy and are eating more simple sugars, you may want to switch towards eating more complex sugars during that time of the day. Pay attention, experiment, and see how you feel so you can make a conscious choice.

If you do not yet know how to read the nutrition label on a package of food, now is a good time to learn. Most adult women should be aiming for a total of 2,000 calories a day and men about 2,500. These numbers are recommended for individuals with their thirty minutes of exercise a day. If you are not getting this exercise you do not need quite as many calories. If you are exercising more you will naturally, need slightly higher calories. To find your ideal calorie goal, it is best to work with a practitioner who will be able to take all of your lifestyle techniques into account. For now, just pay attention to how your body feels and stop when you are filled, not stuffed.

I am always reading all of the different ingredients on nutrition labels. If there are ones I do not know, and do not know how to pronounce, there is a good chance I don't want that unknown thing in my body. I pay attention to the salt content so I know I am getting the right amount daily, as well as the fat content. Now fat content is divided down to saturated fat as well. Saturated and especially trans fats are the ones you want to avoid as much as possible. Depending on the food, if you see these on the label, you may want to just avoid the food all together. For instance, there is no reason for a salad mix to have saturated fats unless there are nuts in it.

For myself, I also pay attention to the protein content in my food. With doing exercise and being a woman, it is important for me to keep my protein levels up so my body can stay strong. I aim to eat about forty grams of protein a day, and most days I am doing good if I get up to thirty. Some individuals will have no trouble with reaching forty or even sixty. This higher level of protein may not be necessary, and if your body is not using it for exercise it is just getting redistributed through your body as fat. Protein foods usually cost more and eating that extra is not only costing you inches on your waist but also dollars in your wallet.

With reading nutrition labels, the more you do it, the more you will know what you personally need to pay attention to. For me it's is the salt and protein content mostly. For others, the amount of carbohydrates they need are just as important as the calorie content. Keep at it and over time you will know more clearly what your body needs and you can choose foods when shopping that will support your body.

Cost is usually the big challenge that you will face with eating healthier. Another large one is taste. It is common that when you start to change the foods you eat you will not like the taste at first. This is because your body has become addicted to sugar and salt. One of the easiest ways to deal with the sugar is to start by adding in more fruit to your diet. Natural sugars will slowly replace your craving for refined sugars. Salt is a different story because usually salt cravings are a craving for minerals that may be missing from our diet.

Two recommendations are to take a multivitamin with microminerals, and to use celtic sea salt or Himalayan pink salt in your cooking. These are colored due to the natural minerals that are in the salts. There are other salts too, but these are common and less expensive than the others. These microminerals will slowly reduce your craving for salty foods which usually lack the actual minerals you are craving them for. If you do not want to add salt to your food, put a pinch into your water. It will give your water some density and you generally will not taste it. If you can taste the salt in your water you either have too much salt in your water or you have been eating too much salt in your diet.

Commonly for individuals who menstruate, cravings will show up through your menstrual cycle. I would recommend following these cravings. Usually your body needs something. If you are craving meat, eat good quality meat. If you are craving sweet, eat the fruits that are sweet. You can make healthy choices that match what you are craving. If you are craving fried food have some sautéed vegetables with a nice heavy olive oil to fulfil your desire for the fat.

If you have multiple people living in the same space, not everyone is going to have the same food requirements. It can be a great allure because even if you have removed your own food temptations, because you have no control over the food of others in your space. Having healthy 'bad foods' is always a good idea. One recommendation for this is having popcorn around, unsalted and unbuttered so you can add only what you want. By itself, popcorn is not a problem for most people and is a super easy and inexpensive treat.

Learning how to cook is often a challenge for people when they are starting to work on their own nourishment. Taking classes in cooking is an easy way to learn more about cooking. It also introduces you to new foods. Community colleges usually have inexpensive cooking classes, and often times higher caliber grocery stores will have free cooking classes to get you into their store. When you are going around grocery stores you will often see little recipe cards. Pick them up. Some stores even have electronic recipe finders. You scan the produce or type in the number and it brings up a variety of recipes using that ingredient. If you buy food you don't know, make sure to write down the correct spelling of the produce. Looking up recipes online is very easy and there are lots of free options available online.

COMMON FOOD COMPLAINTS

DAIRY

Dairy is odd. When I was in basic physiology in college and studying genetic challenges, we often would look at digestion of dairy. When humans are born, they produce enzymes from their genetic code to digest their mother's milk. These enzymes continue to be produced as the child gets older, but as they get older the body starts using a different set of genes to manufacture the enzymes to break down dairy. By about age 16, the genes to make these enzymes are not being produced anymore, and our bodies have greatly reduced capacity to digest dairy products. Different people from different genetic regions continue their production of dairy digesting enzymes for different lengths of time. Only a small genetic group, originating from Northeast Europe, tend to keep their ability to produce dairy digesting enzymes later into life, after high school. Some genetic groups, specifically those originating in Africa, tend to lose their ability to digest dairy at an even younger age and more consistently have observed dairy challenges.

> *But I can digest dairy just fine.*

This is what everyone says until they actually observe themselves. It is true that everyone digests things differently because we all make different enzymes. This is why conscious eating is all the more important to determine if dairy is actually good for you or not. I went two and a half years of experimenting with reduced dairy until I started to actually observe how I would react when I had dairy. I observed that it was specific to different kinds of dairy from different animals, and even different farms and processing techniques.

Now that I know my reaction I can make the decision to have the dairy products or not depending on if I am willing to have the reaction that I know I have. With dairy, many people choose to take enzyme supplements to support the body's natural digestive process. This is a choice you can make. Be aware that this could still not be a cure all for you, and pay attention here as well to know if it is a choice you do want to make.

There are many different kinds of dairy out there and when you target how you react to them it will be very clear what your body can handle. One of the largest differences among dairy products is if it is fermented or not. Fermented dairy includes kefir, real yogurt, cheeses, and sour cream. Fermentation starts the breakdown of lactose sugar by a variety of bacteria. Not only does this reduce the possibility of reaction to the sugars, but the added positive bacteria can support healthy gut flora when eaten.

Non-fermented foods like regular milk, ice cream, and non-fermented yogurts do not have these benefits and can create more problems if ingested by someone who is sensitive to dairy. Sometimes having raw or organic dairy can be better than conventional, non-fermented dairy products. This is generally due to the natural nutrients and enzymes that remain in the milk with less processing.

How do you experience dairy products?

Is your experience different with different dairy products?

Now, not everyone experiences dairy as a sensitivity or an allergy. Some individuals experience dairy as an addiction. What?! Really?! Yes, for some individuals the feeling they get from eating dairy is one they are addicted to. When our bodies get used to having diary and always get inflamed and tight we can get anxious when we do not have this feeling, making us crave dairy even more. This is a challenging habit to break and is not as uncommon as it may sound. Pay attention to this for yourself. It is unfortunate, but it is very common that the food we crave most is one we are addicted to because our bodies are irritated by it in some fashion.

GRAINS

There is so much of a discussion on wheat and gluten these days. So much arguing, too. With all of the different stories out there on if wheat and gluten cause problems, the best method is to test it for yourself. There are people out there with celiac disease, an actual allergy with an immune response to wheat. These are rare cases, and yet many people still report a variety of symptoms associated with foods made with wheat and other gluten containing grains who are not celiac. Celiac is a disease where an individual has an allergy to gluten, rather than a sensitivity or irritation.

My personal experience with gluten containing grains is not that exciting. As a project while in my herbal medicine program, I kept getting told to try to go gluten free for a few weeks to see what would happen. Well the first few times I did this nothing happened. Someone told me then, 'you didn't do it long enough.' So I went a month. And again, 'you didn't do it long enough.' For 3 years, I went on and off gluten, usually buying my alternatives or my glutinous products from Whole Foods, MOM's Organic Market, or other natural food stores.

A few years back I went to visit my parents in Maine, where there is only one Whole Foods Market in the entire state. I tried to stock up but no luck. I had to have gluten most of my meals or I would not have had enough to eat. The food I needed was just not available at the stores or restaurants. Now many people react to gluten with inflamed intestines, aches, headaches, and a variety of other problems. I got mad and depressed all in one go. I was yelling for no good reason at people that did not deserve it. This was not me and something was wrong. Having now found the results of eating gluten, I could more clearly observe when it was happening.

I have since found that I can have some wheat containing products with little problem. I still need to get these foods from the natural food stores, so I just go with the gluten free versions anyways because my reaction is always changing. It could be the processing or the other ingredients, but I now know more clearly my symptoms, so I can make a choice as to what I am going to eat. After paying more attention, the word I have come to use to describe my emotional changes is 'paranoia.' When someone says that they do not have problems with gluten, but are on antidepressants and other mental therapy drugs, I hope they are looking into alternative dietary therapies for their mental wellbeing as well.

Not everyone has a gluten or wheat sensitivity, but if you are not paying attention and having reactions you will not be able to find out what the problem could be. Then you will not have the knowledge you need to make a choice to put the food into your body or not.

Now wheat and gluten are not the only grain problems out there. I do not have personal experience with this one yet, but corn is another up and coming food allergen. Corn is causing even more destructive problems than wheat, primarily because it is in absolutely everything. If you think it is hard to avoid wheat, try to avoid corn. With the high push towards corn syrup over the last decade, corn as an allergen has skyrocketed right along with it. It is another allergen that is often missed but once you know you have it, it can quickly be deadly, like celiac.

Gluten sensitivity often comes about from leaky gut syndrome. Leaky gut syndrome is also one way that a corn allergy can be obtained. How these acquired allergies work is that when the particles get into the body through the leaky intestines, the immune system creates antibodies to tag the particles to be destroyed by the immune system. These tags then remain in the system for future invasions of the particles, which will promote subsequent immune reactions. This is why you do not always react the first time you have something you are allergic to. A great example is what happens when you get stung by a bee. Being celiac is different from this sensitivity, and should be discussed with a professional.

MEAT

Many people make a choice to remove or reduce a variety of animal proteins from their diets. For some, this is an ethical decision, but for others it is because of how their body feels in response to eating the protein. Unfortunately, there are proteins and nutrients that we must have to survive, and if we are not using supplements for these nutrients, we need to eat animal proteins. I am very much an advocate of choosing what you put into your body through how you feel in response to it. Often, a more vegetarian regime feels best for most people. However, for those who are vegetarian, animal proteins every so often can truly support a healthy lifestyle. Animal protein can reduce the need of supplementation, which can have its own challenges.

During menstruation, having red meat can be necessary prior to menstruation to build up the blood with added iron. While there are many vegetarian sources of iron and other blood building nutrients, they are harder to digest and absorb when they come from plant sources. Finding a balance between animal and non-animal protein sources and seeing what works best for you is the way to go.

Fish and shellfish proteins may serve as an alternative for some required nutrients but allergies to these are very common and should be taken seriously. Oily fish such as salmon and sardines, are highly suggested when additional oil needs to be added to your food regimen. This is why fish oils supplements are so popular.

It is also important to note that there are a variety of new diseases that are altering how we interact with animal proteins. One of these, a relatively new tick born disease from a Lone Star Tick, actually prompts allergic reactions when different kinds of meats are digested. These reactions are just as serious as shellfish allergies, requiring immediate injections with an epinephrine-pen in response to a reaction. Take care in observing what you are eating in regards to these allergies. In some cases, there is not choice in what to eat, because death can be a quick result of eating these foods if you are allergic to them.

OTHER COMMON RESPONSE FOODS

Nightshades

The idea of poisonous nightshades is familiar to most of us. This plant family, common in many parts of the world, has many poisonous species. When the first colonizers arrived in the Americas they were introduced to a few of the non-poisonous varieties such as tomatoes. Other non-poisonous varieties include potatoes, peppers, and eggplants. While most people do not have sensitivities the fruits of these plants, because of their close relativity to poisonous varieties, sensitivity is not unheard of. One of the symptoms that can go with sensitivity to nightshades are increased acid production in the stomach, causing heart burn and similar. Peppers will also sometimes have bacteria growing on them that can cause an upset stomach. Washing does not always remove these, but it is best to always wash your vegetables anyways.

Roses

Sensitivities to fruits from the rose family are even more uncommon to those of the nightshade family. Examples of fruits would be apples, peaches, and pears. The sensitivity to these fruits are more common when they are raw. Cooking and adding herbs that support digestive function like cinnamon can help one to digest these fruits more effectively. Problems digesting these and other fruits often show in the in bowels via increased liquid in the stool.

Poison ivy family

I was often told through herbal medicine school that the family containing poison ivy contained a variety of foods that people have a tendency to be sensitive to. Poison ivy is, in my experience, a plant that not everyone is allergic to when they touch it. I am one of the lucky people and I do not react to the plant if I handle it. I have once gotten the oils of the plant directly into my blood stream and I had a reaction as a result. There is a tendency for people who are allergic to this plant to also have sensitivities to <u>mango</u> and <u>cashews</u>. This sensitivity is not always going to be to all three of these plants but if you have sensitivities to two of them I would pay close attention to the third when you ingest it.

A side note to think about. It is common for an individual to just be allergic to poison ivy. It is common for an individual to just be allergic to cashews. It is much rarer for an individual just to be allergic to mango. I recently found that when this is the case, it is not generally due to the poison ivy family allergy, but rather an allergy to latex. If you are having allergy symptoms due to mango, please seek a professional allergist and be tested for a latex allergy. This can be a serious allergy if not appropriately managed, so take care and look into it now.

THE CHOICE IS YOURS

Remember, conscious eating is all about empowering yourself to make the choices you feel will help you feel better, to give you the energy you need and the nutrients to allow your body to function properly. It allows you to decide when to have things that may be somewhat detrimental to your wellbeing. I hope that through your own exploration you will come to find what your own interactions with them will teach you in regards to what works best with your body.

What other areas of your life can you use this observation and conscious choice technique?

CHAPTER 14: STRESS REDUCTION TECHNIQUES

Homework Assignment 11

Observe and record the following for a week.

What caused you stress today?
What actually happened? What was the phenomena?
What choices could you make so this would not stress you?
What choices could you make to remove this challenge?
Would these changes serve you?

How do you define stress?

The word stress specifically refers to the importance we attach to something. 'I stress that this is important,' is a good example to remind ourselves of this. Emphasizing that something is prominent, putting physical or other pressure onto a person or idea, is stress. While these definitions may not exactly resonate with your experience, it does make us think about the cause of our stressful feelings. Stress, in the physiological sense, is a specific response to a stimulus, such as fear or pain, that alters our normal physiological balance. Anxiety is similar; a feeling of distress or uneasiness caused by fear, danger, or misfortune. It can also be apprehension or eagerness towards a situation.

Feelings of stress and anxiety appear differently for different people. Often we get used to feeling 'stressed' and forget what normal feels like. This is not uncommon. Starting to pay attention to your body and how it reacts in different settings is key to determining what is actually causing you stress. Then you can make adjustments to lower your stress response. Using our conscious techniques that we practiced in our conscious eating chapter, we can see our bodies responses in a different light.

Let's check in with our bodies right now for practice!

How are your legs and feet feeling right now?

How does your pelvic region feel right now?

How does your abdomen feel right now?

How do your hands and arms feel right now?

How does your chest feel right now?

How does your neck region feel right now?

How does your head feel right now?

Are any of these feelings ones that you associate with stress?

When you feel stress or anxiety, where does it show up in your body? What are some words to describe the feeling?

Some individuals tend to get tightness in their neck and shoulders when they feel stressed. Others get nervous stomachs. When I am in an emergency situation, sometimes I have even felt the adrenaline rushing from my heart towards my extremities. Starting to see the signs of when you are stressed is the first step to working with the stressful situation to reduce the impact that it has on you.

Many of us know that the stress feeling is a response humans have evolved to have. It is part of our fight or flight mechanism. When we sense danger, our neurons release cytokines that cause a chain reaction causing our responses to stress. Stress can be due to visual, mental, physical, or emotional experiences. This reaction occurs any time we understand a situation to be threatening to our wellbeing or safety. Over time, it can become a chronic state of being alert, and trying to inhibit the reaction can cause even more damage. This can lead to self-destructive behaviors such as overworking, overeating, and thrill seeking behavior in an attempt to maintain the feeling we perceive to be normal, a state of stress.

WHAT IS STRESS DOING TO US?

The biochemical mechanism in our body that is our stress response is what is called a negative feedback loop. As our stress hormone, cortisol, gets higher in our body it reduces the production of the molecules that cause cortisol to be created in the first place. For some individuals, cortisol is produced continuously due to long term exposure to stressors and the feedback loop does not shut off.

This is not uncommon today. We become desensitized and can no longer shut down cortisol production because we are constantly experiencing stress. When this is occurring, the only way to shut down the loop is to use our higher brain centers to consciously reduce our stress levels. This comes from practicing making new memories where stress is not included.

Are there memories that cause you stress when you think about them?

What stressors have you experienced that have led to you getting sick?

A relatively new field of science, psychoneuroimmunology, describes to us how our nervous system and immune system are all connected. This is greatly important to everyone who has ever gotten sick. We all know that college students when they come home for breaks tend to get sick and again during midterms and finals. This is due to the stress they experience which can greatly lower their immune system's ability to keep them healthy. High levels of cortisol can directly cause death of T cells, important immune cells in our bodies. Short term stress can increase our immune system's function but most of us have not experienced 'short term' stress for many years. Long term, chronic stress, lasting more than a week will start to reduce your immune systems function on all levels. It is also not uncommon to get Functional Hypothyroidism when stress has been high for long periods of time. This has its own set of symptoms that can alter our digestion, skin and hair health, mental capacity, blood pressure, and many other things.

What things have caused you to have a 'nervous stomach'?

While it may not be intuitive to most of us, we do also have nervous tissue in our digestive system. This is why we get nervous stomachs before presentations, and why when we are upset we tend to either crave food or lose our appetite all together. This could be one of the possible reasons behind Inflammatory Bowel Syndrome (IBS). IBS is a general inflammation of the digestive system causing a variety of problems such as bowel movement challenges, challenges absorbing nutrients, and absorbing a higher number of potential allergen and toxic substances through the digestive tract. This theory suggests that stress alters our nervous system in our digestive tract, irritating our immune system causing the inflammation associated with IBS. Though this may not be the cause for everyone, reducing your stress level can be one possible treatment to add to your regime.

What symptoms do you experience when you are stressed?

In the digestive tract, stress can cause more stomach acid production and cause the formation of ulcers in the intestines. The pancreas generally regulates our blood sugar, but when stressed, its ability to perform this function is lowered, which can alter our blood sugar and, in response, our moods. This is especially important to keep in mind for those with diabetes and with a family history of diabetes.

It is not uncommon to eat when stressed. Food is often a comfort for us and we choose to indulge ourselves a little when we are not feeling great. While this is fine in moderation, when we just sit and eat food because we are bored or need to block out the stress that is around us, this kind of eating is not great for us.

Generally, when this is happening, we reach for the foods we already know our body does not agree with. The best choice you can make here is to choose foods that will reduce your stress and support your wellness rather than picking something that will not help you. You can also choose to exercise. Another way to help yourself is by drinking more water in place of food to calm your appetite and give you something to keep doing to occupy your mind.

For some of us food itself can be a stressor. The most obvious reason for this is because some people are afraid of weight they may gain from food. It can also be a stressor if you have any food allergies or sensitivities. Our conscious eating chapter takes a deeper look at empowering you if you have food sensitivities to make the choices you need to make, and want to make, to support your wellness around food.

If food is a stressor for you, it can be a challenge to approach food at all. It can just add even more stress to your life. Start with experimenting with what you feel comfortable with, and what you are used to. When looking at how food affects you it is great to try new things, but do not feel like you need to remove your favorite foods from your diet because someone told you to. Remember, the choice is yours and removing something you like from your diet may be more mentally detrimental than physically beneficial.

When we are stressed, our heart rates are one of the easiest things to experience and pay attention to. Adrenaline, released when you are stressed, increases both your heart rate and blood pressure. We usually can feel our heart rate increase in a similar fashion to when we have exerted ourselves with exercise. For some this can be good but for most of us, a higher heart rate and blood pressure can mean serious consequences that can even lead to heart attacks.

Healthy individuals with low stress and frequent exercise tend to have heart rates under 60bpm. Over time, exercise will lower your heart rate as your cardiovascular system strengthens. This will reduce the negative effects that increased blood pressure and heart rate due to stress will have on your body because your body is stronger.

Do you notice a change in your stress experience with exercise?

Having an overall healthy and well body helps support how you adapt to stressful situations. For example, having antioxidants in your diet reduces inflammation, exercising to reduce your heart rate and strengthening your muscles and cardiopulmonary systems, sleeping so that you can process daily events - all of these things support your wellness, allowing you to have a healthy and well body able to deal with daily stressors.

When we are stressed, we produce inducible Nitric Oxide Synthase (iNOS). iNOS is used by our immune system to kill pathogens and keep us safe. When it is raised and no pathogens are present, it can actually start to damage our bodies. This is one area where antioxidants work to reduce oxidative damage from various sources in our body.

Stress can directly affect the urogenital system of both men and women. When stressed, vaginal infections become more common, and becoming erect can be challenging. All genders experience lower sexual desire when they are experiencing high levels of stress, and some may not even release eggs on their monthly cycle when stressed. If you have recently given birth, with high stress levels, your milk production can also be reduced. Menopause symptoms also tend to be worse with high levels of stress. And stress can increase testosterone, which in high levels is neurotoxic and will start to cause additional nervous system damage.

Write a list of the top 10 things that are important to you in your life.

Now circle the ones that cause you stress in your life.

145

Generally, we only become stressed around events or situations that we have defined as being important to us. If they were not important, we would not worry about them. This is a conscious choice we make regarding our stress response. You do not have to worry about things. Upset is optional and you can choose to let things go. It takes some practice to be able to do this.

DEALING WITH YOUR STRESS AND ANXIETY

Most of us 'freak out' when we are stressed, and it can cause us to create difficult situations for ourselves that we may not otherwise get into. A very common occurrence of this is road rage. When you aren't having a good day, you are more likely to cut someone off or not stop for a stop sign. Being frustrated, stressed, or anxious about something can take a lot of our attention away from the other things we normally do, such as treating others with consideration of their feelings. While this is not always the case, it is important to recognize when your feelings involving a particular situation are impacting other areas of your life.

What was an occurrence when your feelings about a situation took control of you in another situation, causing upset there?

What could you have done to keep the events separate from each other or to let go of the upset so it would not affect your reactions to other events?

While it is not usually a cure all, this is an excellent time to use the practice 'Yes, Yes, NOW' that we discussed in the behavior change chapter. Could you let it go? Would you let it go? When? -or- Could you? Would you? When? Can you let go of your road rage for 15 minutes to have a meeting with your boss, or to say hello to your children when you first get home?

JOURNALING ABOUT STRESS

The best way to start to target the specific things that cause you stress is to journal frequently about your day. Many irritations cause us stress. Some are our job and family. Other irritations are harder to observe, like having to go to the bank or talking to a specific person at work. Journaling can help you focus on what these irritations are, so you can work to find an active way of dealing with them.

Looking at the phenomena, at what was actually said and done, not what was implied or how you interpreted what happened, can be difficult at first. Journaling can help encourage you to process and interpret the events from another viewpoint. When you look just at the phenomena, big things seem much smaller than they first were. The phenomena can help to put things into perspective for us.

Last year I was at an event, and I had a huge pile of things I had to complete on a deadline. I was completely stressed out. Things were wrapping up for the evening, and I was lucky enough to have won an award on one of my projects. I started to feel upset at myself, like I had not been successful. I took some time to go relax and look at all of the things I had accomplished through the day. I began to see that things were not that bad, even though I was feeling terrible. I had what is known as adrenal fatigue, when your adrenal gland has produced so many stress hormones that your body starts to go into a depressed state, generally a place of full body tiredness. I was able to spend the evening relaxing to reduce the hormones in my system, so that the next day I could be my normal chipper self and keep going.

Looking at each individual thing you feel upset or stressed about can be important because, sometimes, you can use problem solving skills to feel better and less stressed. Other times you can look at new possibilities of how you can act differently in a situation to reduce your stress response, or to prevent the problem from becoming stressful in the first place.

As we have been journaling as we go through this guidebook you have probably come across a variety of choices you make that lead to the same result consistently. Similarly, you may notice experiences with your body and have learned what changes in activity can make these things stop or increase, as desired. When you find a symptom that you can change, remember it. This is a tool. I know that when my skin starts to get dry, I have not been listening to my thirst reflex telling me to drink more water. I know that when I have dryer skin I tend to get sick more so I better listen up and drink that water or risk getting sick. We all have little things like this that our body tells us but we forget about. Journaling helps us to keep track of these details we may otherwise forget.

What are five of your symptom reminder tools?

STRESS PREVENTION TOOLS

For most of us, we like to prevent upsets from occurring by avoiding them in the first place. This can be a great temporary solution, but speaking in long term, if your stressor is still in your life it can be painful and challenging. So do not stop here. After observing your situation, you will be able to start to see how it affects you more clearly and how your life could be improved without the challenging situation. By avoiding or removing the challenge it will be easier to see how it alters your mood and stress levels. This is when you are able to take your choice to move on, or hold onto your challenge. The choice is yours to hold onto your stress or work towards wellness.

If you cannot remove your stressor long term, practicing 'Could you? Would you? When?' is a way to slowly increase your ability to deal with the stressor. Take it just one step at a time. It is hard to let go of things that irritate us. Often we become attached to the feeling it offers our body. We start to think of anxiety as normal, when it is not. It is hard to begin to see that it is not normal to feel that way, because observing the effect is the hardest part.

Again, journaling and talking it out with another person is a great way to target the stressors you are experiencing. For my most recent upset and stressor, what I needed to do was basically research myself. I was finding I had fear regarding a few specific people for unclear reasons. By releasing my fear and letting that go by not dwelling on it, I was able to talk to those people and learn more about them, enough to find that my fear was completely invalid I did not need to hold onto it anymore. In this instance, communication was all that it took me to release a problem that had been in my life for a whole year, and had been holding me back from new possibilities.

REDUCING STRESS

Exercise is a great way to reduce your experience of stress. When you exercise the hormone oxytocin is released. This hormone offers a feeling of security, contentment, and bonding to the experience and to those around you. This same hormone is released during breast feeding and hugging your friends and loved ones. This hormone makes us feel happy. Exercise also encourages your blood to be directed towards your muscles and away from your digestive system and brain. This is part of the flight or fight mechanism. Lucky for us, many of our stressors just come from thinking about them over and over again. Exercise can actually reduce your thinking about your stressors, which, long term, reduces their effect on you. Often we end up socializing when we exercise, which also supports stress reduction through bonding with others. Often this leads to talking out the things that are causing us upset while exercising or socializing with others.

In addition to social support, having repetition and stability in your life can be a large factor of reducing stress. Having a set schedule of work, waking and sleeping, fun, exercise, and other activities can be important. Consistency and stability by themselves reduce our stress. A schedule is also the easiest way to make sure you are incorporating other wellness and stress reducing behaviors in your life. Taking a break, having a massage, going for a swim, all of these things are also great ways to reduce your stress level. Take a day at the spa, go tinker in the garage on a project, have fun and find some time for yourself.

Here is a sample schedule including all of the wellness related activities included in this guidebook, with enough time to prepare and cook all of your own meals, exercise, get enough sleep, time for relaxation, work, and spiritual activities (when shifted to meet your time needs). Having this kind of basic outline can be helpful so you know you really do have time to do everything. Even with an hour of family time, cleaning, and spiritual activities every day, there is still at least two hours of personal time each day.

```
6am: Waking Ritual      12: Lunch           8pm: Personal Time
6:30: Exercise          1-5: Work           9pm: Self Care
7am: Breakfast          6pm: Family Time        and Relaxation
8-Noon: Work            7pm: Dinner         10pm: Sleep
```

While this is a busy looking schedule for some, it does have a large amount of relaxation time and free time in it every day. On the weekends or on days you are not working, there is even more free time. During these times I recommend taking the time to do your errands, prepare food for the week, and similar things. Don't feel that you have to stick to this exact schedule. At **www.thedancingherbalist.com** you can find a worksheet to help you develop a regular schedule that will work for you.

Empowering yourself to make these commitments to stress reduction and wellness is challenging, and being able to say 'NO' and 'I don't know' to events and questions that come up can be a real skill to have. Those of us with busy schedules tend to have a hard time saying no to people, and having so much on our plates eventually will run us dry. Practice saying no, even just to yourself. While many people will feel insulted when you turn them down, it should not be a reflection on you, but rather their expectations of you as we discussed in chapter 12.

You have control over your actions, not the actions of others. Practice empowering yourself to say no when you are asked to do something that may encourage stress in your life. The first few times you say 'no' to doing something can be challenging. Remember you are taking control and you don't have to do something you do not want to do. You get to choose everything about your life. Don't forget that!

It can also serve you to practice saying you do not know something. This goes along with practicing saying 'no.' As we discussed in our chapter 12, it is often hard for individuals to reduce expectations so if you cannot meet the expectations someone is putting on you, let them know. This can release a lot of stress that is put upon you.

Even though these two techniques may lower your stress, it is important to remember that sometimes stress can fuel us to keep going.

Life is always moving and changing. Without movement, there is no life. If you are struggling with opposition to something, practice drawing a larger circle. In a circle, you can be next to something or across from it. In a larger circle, something that was opposite of you becomes closer to your side. You do not need to be in opposition, think of the problem through a larger framework. You may be arguing on how to get a project done but you are all working together for the same goal of the project and that is what you really want to all accomplish. You can't skip the many upsets that happen. You have to work with them and go with the flow. Your dog may be scratching at the door and upsetting your schedule, but if you don't get off the couch to let him outside you will have even more upset. Keep life and its conflicts moving.

Beyond anything else I have tried for reducing stress, I have found that consistent meditation is the best treatment. There are many kinds of meditation practices. We talked about three different breathing techniques for meditation in chapter 7, and these can be helpful for stress reduction. Meditations are helpful when falling asleep because they reduce our mental chatter and help us focus on calming our minds and bodies to prepare for sleep. Consistent practice of meditating calms our minds and bodies through the day and reduces our chances of becoming upset, lashing out, and stressing over things.

What things will you be adding to your life to reduce your stress?

What things will you be removing from your life to reduce your stress?

How will you alter your interactions with others to reduce the stress in your life?

CHAPTER 15: COMMON HYDRATION CHALLENGES

Homework Assignment 12

Choose one flavored water at the end of this chapter and choose to make this. Substitute one non-water drink you have a day with this flavored water or tea for one week. In your journal, record how easy or hard it was for you to make this change. Would you continue to substitute your beverages for water? What would make it easier for you to do this?

How are you doing at staying hydrated? Now that you have had time to practice, let's look at some of the common challenges there are to staying hydrated and how you can overcome them.

Water temperature

We talked about this briefly when discussing the properties of water, but the temperature of water will greatly matter when we start to increase our hydration levels. It actually takes our body energy to warm up water to a temperature that it can be absorbed. Because of this, warm and room temperature liquids are much better for us to drink. Singers know this and enjoy warm water because cold water will shrink the vocal cords and it takes time and energy to re-warm our system. While you can drink cold liquids and still become hydrated, if you are trying to maximize the efficiency of the liquids you drink you should drink them at room temperature or warmer.

So coffee and tea are great then, right?

Unfortunately, there is another problem with coffee and tea that we have not discussed at all. Coffee and tea, green, black, and other non-herbal teas all contain what are called tannins. Some herbal teas also contain tannins but most do not. These molecules 'tan' our digestive tract and actually bind the proteins of the cells together, making it harder to actually absorb water. At low levels this is not a large problem but when you are drinking large amounts of coffee and black tea, it can actually reduce the amount of water you are absorbing. This is one reason that when you drink coffee first thing in the morning it is common to have a bowel movement. The increased fluids in the bowels prompts evacuation. It is recommended that for every cup of tea or coffee you drink you then drink an additional cup of water that you would not normally drink.

So, how much water should I drink?

How much water you should drink is debatable. I take the route of paying attention to all of my hydration signs to see if I need to drink more.

This is what I recommend rather than saying a number. There are individuals who swear that you need to drink an entire gallon a day of water to stay healthy. That is an awful lot of water, and if you are a person with low blood pressure, drinking this much water can actually be detrimental. I do see benefit from drinking minimally 8 cups of water a day for most individuals, if not more. Eight cups, half a gallon, two Nalgene bottles, and four generic plastic water bottles are all the same amount of water. However, once you start to factor in movement and sweating you should be adding more to this amount of water.

I once decided to drastically increase my water and aimed for drinking the gallon a day. That is sometimes considered an upper limit for how much water to drink in a day. When I first woke up I drank four cups before doing anything. When you drink that much water in one sitting your stomach feels stretched out, and it is. While I felt that for the first few days this was energizing me, after a few days I began to feel lightheaded as I went through my day. However, some people this high level of water is great, and can clear skin problems, give energy and other benefits to the drinker. Drinking water is another practice that is important to find what works best for you, to get all of the benefits and fewer of the negatives.

How much water you will need to drink will also depend on your size. Taller and larger people in general have more blood, and to keep their blood and all of their tissues well hydrated they need to drink considerably more. This extra water is especially important in taller people who should generally have a higher blood pressure to get blood higher when circulating. Smaller people may need less water but for the most part **more water is better** and should be reached for.

I am drinking lots of water but all it does is give me diarrhea.

There are a few things to think about when this is happening. First, is it actually diarrhea or are your stools just looser? If they are just looser, do not worry about it. This is good, it will help to clear out your colon of matter that may sometimes get stuck there. Flip back to the Bristol stool chart and check it out. However, if you are having serious diarrhea, do go see a doctor as this should not be happening. Some individuals struggle with absorbing water. When this is happening for me I find that adding a touch of a nice celtic sea salt to my water will help me absorb it.

Flavor

One major problem a lot of people have when trying to get more water when they first start out is that it doesn't taste good. For the most part, water has a neutral taste, and when all we are used to drinking is high sugar drinks, water can take some time to adjust to the taste. When you are transitioning I have a few great recommendations.

Let's start on the path of highest resistance. If you are having sodas like Coke and Pepsi, or even Sierra Mist start here. When you transition away from these high sugar drinks, it can be hard to skip to a non-carbonated drink first. I recommend either investing in a soda machine or plain carbonated water and then add 100% fruit juices to your drink. When you buy 100% fruit juices, you will see they are expensive. That is why we dilute them either in regular or sparkling water. This makes it fun as well. You get to do your own drink mixing. Try different fruits. My favorites are cranberries, pomegranates, and blueberry juice. You can also find things like strawberry and mango if you look hard enough. The fruit 'nectars' that you may find are not as good since they are higher in sugar than sodas, even when you do dilute them with sparkling water, so I advise against using those.

When I was transitioning from drinking soda to drinking mostly water, this step was crucial on my path to wellness. It took me months but once I was finally getting the hang of making these drinks and enjoying them, I started to enjoy them more than other sodas. Even now I make them every so often because they are a great treat.

Once you are starting to cut down on sugar, it is easy to find low sugar things to add to water so it tastes better. Some of these things include drink mixes. Now, drink mixes are generally high in sugar, but over time your tastes will become accustomed to having more water and less drink mix in your cup as you reduce the amount of mix you use. I like this because drink mixes let you control how much sugar you put into your water. I like to take a cup of water and add drink mix to it rather than starting with a set amount of mix in my cup. This way I only add as much as I need.

A great nutritious drink mix brand is Oxylent. A lot of people go for Emergency C, but, personally, I do not want to drink that every day. Oxylent was originally designed for individuals going through chemotherapy who were struggling to stay hydrated. Oxylent carbonates the water and also provides a full days' worth of vitamins in your cup. Oxylent can be purchased by many pharmacies by special order. There are other brands as well, and they can all help you drink more water by adding a bit of flavor and bubbles to the mix. Another sweetener option is to use honey or maple syrup in place of granular sugar. These sweeteners are closer to their natural state allowing our bodies to more easily compensate for their adjustments to our blood sugar levels.

Often in stores we will see vitamin waters and other flavored waters. These can be all right but look at the labels. A lot of times these will also be high in sugars and other things your body may be sensitive to. That is all right. You can make your own flavored waters at home for a fraction of the price. Take some fruits, herbs, or vegetables if you'd like, and cut them into slices, put them into a jar and add water to fill the jar. This is great for kids because they love to see the colors of the fruits in their jars, and is refreshing in the summer. If you search online for 'homemade fruit water' you get a lot of great recipe ideas for this. Here are a few of my favorites.

For all of these recipes, slice the food, cover with ice, and pour water over the food and ice. Add straw and enjoy! You can also pour hot water over it if you want a fruit tea. You can always add more water after you have drunk what is in your jar to re-use the fruits.

Citrus
1 orange, 1 lime, and 1 lemon and put them into 2-4 quart size jars.

Lime mint
1-2 limes and 3 fresh mint leaves for 1 quart jar.

Raspberry Lime
1 lime and ½ cup raspberries for 1 quart jar.

Orange Carrot
Slice 1 orange and grate 1 large carrot for 2 quart jars.

Other fruits and vegetables that go well in these infused waters are cucumber, strawberries, melons, as well as herbs like lemon balm, basil, and a touch of lavender. Watermelon can even be popped in the blender and made into ice cubes in the freezer to drop in water by themselves. This also works well when you are out to dinner and are trying to have more water. Usually restaurants will offer you lemon for your water. Go for it, ask for more lemon if you would like to make it even stronger in your water. With trying these transitional beverages, you will be on your way in no time to having more water in your daily life.

What kinds of flavored water would you like to try?

When will you make your flavored water?

Have you found techniques that you can implement in the next day to increase your hydration?

What techniques are you going to use to make your water intake sustainable for the long term?

What benefits are you going to receive from increasing your water intake?

CHAPTER 16: THE CAUSE IS INFLAMMATION

Inflammation is your body's reaction to just about anything that your body believes is dangerous. This includes physical damage, emotional damage, pathogens such as bacteria and viruses, foreign objects like food or plant allergens, and can even result when you have not let your body heal with proper amounts of sleep. Not only does inflammation cause all of these things, it can also be **the cause** of many of these things as well. Inflammation is complicated. Let's start by looking at what happens when one of these 'inflammatory stimuli' enters our body's system.

There are five signs of inflammation we experience in our body due to these causes. The signs include heat, redness, swelling, pain, and loss of function in the affected area. Pay attention to these signs to notice how your inflammation changes over time.

ACUTE INFLAMMATION

Acute, or temporary, inflammation happens right when your body detects something is wrong. When detection occurs, your body sends leukocytes, a white blood cell, to the region of detection. This is done through altering the blood pressure so that the leukocytes in the blood can be directed accordingly. The extra blood and fluid, at the location of detection, is what we usually refer to as inflammation, the puffiness of the skin. Individual cells absorb more fluid and become larger, expanding gaps between cells so the leukocytes can actually get to the problem by escaping the blood stream.

Leukocytes will specifically attack pathogens. They detect the problem and release antibodies to encourage white blood cells to come take care of the specific problem. White blood cells then work to kill or remove the pathogens present. When there is physical damage, not a pathogen, the additional blood flow supports the healing process by bringing molecules the body uses to heal. This is why the body says "Damage? Inflammation!" Inflammation will take care of the problem, whether it is physical damage, pathogen, or allergen.

When there is physical damage, fibrous tissue can grow to try to cover up the injury. The molecules to do this are delivered with the increased blood supply. This fibrous tissue, if not removed and replaced

159

by the body's tissue generation methods, can register to the body systems if 'something is wrong.' If this occurs, it can lead to chronic inflammation. Similarly, if a pathogen is not fully taken care of, killed or removed by white blood cells, it can also lead to chronic inflammation.

CHRONIC INFLAMMATION

The process of destroying pathogens and allergens includes releasing a variety of molecules that are toxic in hopes of destroying these invaders. Unfortunately, these toxic substances tend to cause damage to our own tissues in the process. Our bodies sometimes will respond to its own inflammatory response with an even larger inflammatory response, causing even more damage. This kind of cycle is how our bodies get into a constant state of inflammation, chronic inflammation. Chronic inflammation includes, but is not limited to, arthritis, asthma, atherosclerosis, dermatitis, or chondritis and just about any other term you have ever heard ending in '-itis,' meaning an inflammatory condition.

When we have active inflammation, tissue damage, and have been trying to heal for weeks or more, we have entered into the stage of chronic inflammation. The healing process itself here shifts because there is now a balance where the healing process is causing just as much damage as it is repairing because of the damaging effects of inflammation. These damaging effects are from reactive oxygen and nitrogen molecules, proteases, cytokines, and arachidonic acid. The same immune cells that create these, also create growth factors and angiogenesis factors which stimulate blood flow and the healing of tissues.

While cytokines can cause damage at the site of the problem, they, along with the other healing and damaging molecules, can travel through the blood to other parts of the body as well. As they travel they commonly will induce a fever, raising the body's temperature in an attempt to kill pathogens. Cytokines will also increase protein levels in the blood in an attempt to bring healing proteins to the damaged area. Unfortunately, this increase in protein is associated with various heart problems, including, but not limited to, strokes. There is also an increase in release of leukocytes from bone marrow with increased cytokine levels.

This can be concerning, as it will lower our 'reserve pool' for the next time we are sick. This is one reason that immunocompromised individuals are in constant danger of getting a serious illness from even a small infection - they have no reserves.

What inflammation symptoms have you experienced?

Have you recorded any symptoms associated with inflammation in your previous wellness journals?

Do you experience any chronic problems associated with inflammation? What do you think was the cause?

CAUSES OF INFLAMMATION

There is a wide variety of things that can cause inflammation in our body. We can roughly separate the causes into three categories: infection, irritation, and injury. When we discuss our immune system we commonly think about infections and the impact these have on us.

Infections can be bacterial, viral, fungal, and even some parasites. Bacteria are single celled organisms, and often form groups such as the plaque on our teeth. They can be both internal, such as with a cold, or they can be skin infections. Viral infections, like the flu and HIV, hijack our cells to reproduce themselves. They insert their DNA into our cells. This is what makes them so problematic; they hide in our own cells.

Fungal infections can happen internally, but we most commonly think of yeast infections in the urogenital system. We always have fungus on our body, but sometimes one species can take over. What we want is a balance, just like with healthy bacteria found on and in our entire body. Parasites, such as worms and malaria, most affect our body by eating up our essential nutrients and energy sources. They lower our energy and may live in us for ages before we know it. Some, like worms, are easy to get rid of, but others are not and can easily lead to chronic inflammation such as in Lyme disease.

Irritations that stimulate our immune system are our allergens. Allergens can get into our body a few different ways. They can be absorbed through the mucosa in our nose and respiratory tract, absorbed through our skin, or absorbed through our digestive tract. In order to have an irritation or an allergic reaction to something, it must get into our body through one of these pathways. We communicate with the world through these paths and we are exposed to everything either by eating, breathing, or touching. Getting sick through our respiratory system is common for all of us; this is how we get colds and flus and usually react to seasonal allergens.

We have all heard of someone getting a bee sting and swelling up like a balloon. This is a classic acute inflammation case, but we can have more chronic inflammation in our skin as well. These are our eczemas and psoriasis, chronic inflammation often due to irritations either on our skin or systemic through our whole body. As mentioned earlier in this guidebook, inflammatory bowel disease (IBD or IBS) is becoming very common. It is becoming more accepted that the process of this happening is through chronic inflammation in the body opening up larger spaces between cells in the digestive tract. When this happens, molecules that are not supposed to be absorbed, are absorbed, and they stimulate an even worse inflammatory reaction specific to the digestive tract.

Injuries our body experience are usually hard to miss. We cut our hand when slicing vegetables. We break out leg in a fall down the stairs. We have surgery for something. These injuries all cause inflammation so that our bodies can heal. Usually we heal nicely from injuries, but sometimes they can turn into chronic inflammation. This is the case with chronic back pain which usually has an initial injury associated with it. There can be other injuries and damage going inside our body we may not be aware of. Injuries and tissue damage including cancer, which can be very hard to detect even with modern technology. They all cause inflammation.

This is everything that causes inflammation right? Most of these things are not in our control, and we cannot change whether or not we are exposed to the irritants, illnesses, and accidental tissue damage. This is not true though because the different wellness inputs can cause inflammation. A good one to consider is movement. The way we get stronger is by exercising enough to cause tissue damage. Through the healing process we become stronger. We also become inflamed at the same time. This can lead to all of the challenges with inflammation we are discussing in this chapter.

Some of our food choices can also cause inflammation. Meat consumption in high amounts can promote inflammation in our entire body. This is not only because of the high levels of protein, but also because of the type of protein and the energy it takes to break meat down in our bodies. Our bodies don't recognize plants as 'invading pathogens,' but animal proteins are another matter. This is not the case for everyone, but animal proteins can cause inflammation in our bodies. Some people also have foods they are sensitive to and cause irritations in our digestive tract. We talked a little about dairy and wheat in our conscious eating chapter. While these two are common irritants they are by no means the only ones. This is why observing how your body reacts to food is important to not have negative reactions to the things you add to your body.

Is that everything? Nope. In our chapter on stress we also saw that stress and our thoughts can also affect our immune system. Stress lowers our body's ability to fight an infection. What this means is that while we are stressed we may not actually have as bad an inflammatory reaction. This sounds great! Short term it is; this is our fight or flight response, and how we are able to deal with our problems quickly without our immune response getting in the way. However, it means that the healing and actual fighting of infections is put off, and can be made even worse in the meantime.

Now that we know most of the different causes of inflammation, let's look at your experiences with these inflammation inputs. If you list out all possibilities, you will start to see patterns of frequent inflammation pathways in your own body. This will be helpful for you to be able to target the causes of the inflammation you experience, so that you can make changes to prevent this inflammation from becoming chronic.

How frequently do you get colds or flus? (Approximate days a year) How has this affected you?

Do you have any immune compromising infections, such as Mononucleosis (mono), HIV/AIDS, or Lyme disease? How has this affected you?

Have you ever had any parasitic infections? How has this affected you?

Have you experienced fungal overgrowths? How has this affected you?

Do you have any known allergens? How do they affect you?

Do you have any symptoms of allergens or other irritations related to your skin, respiratory, or digestive systems?

Have you ever had any traumatic physical injury? How has this affected you?

Do you exercise regularly and have associated inflammation? How has this affected you?

Are there foods that you eat that cause you upset and inflammation? How do they affect you?

Overall, do you think you experience a lot of inflammation from these causes?

What does the inflammation you experience feel and look like to you in relation to these causes?

WHAT DOES INFLAMMATION AFFECT

A lot of the things that cause inflammation can also be affected and made worse because of the inflammation. An example of inflammation all are likely familiar with is the experience of having a stuffy nose when you have a cold, particularly when you just can't seem to get the fluid out. A stuffy nose and a fever are common inflammatory symptoms. This one simple symptom can lead to inflammation and damage in our whole body. In our circulatory system, cells swell and allow gaps, leaking irritants into the space between cells. The heart may become inflamed and experience stress from increased blood pressure. Both of these things can cause even more inflammation due to irritants and stress.

In our muscles and joints, inflammation will cause even more damage, causing pain, additional swelling, pressure, and in some cases, restriction of function. When your body just feels like a dull ache, and you don't really feel like moving, this is inflammation in your muscles. Nerves are closely associated with our muscles as they promote the actual contractions of muscles. Inflammation can damage and break down the insulation around our nerve cells thereby reducing the ability of our nerves to work. This causes contractions, and responses to other stimuli like pain. This is why when you have an old cut you may not feel pain there any longer; your nerves have been damaged. This can lead to even more damage when we cannot feel pain in response to trauma. Again, all of this damage from inflammation can cause even more inflammation.

The digestive system is where herbalists personally see the largest effects of inflammation due to IBS and related conditions. Inflammation is more problematic in the intestines than the inflammation in the blood vessels (where the irritants escaping circulation are already in the body) because irritants that get in through inflamed intestine are not supposed to be in our body in the first place. When this occurs, it is anyone's guess as to what will happen, because it is not something our bodies have evolved to deal with. We did not evolve to deal with the petrochemicals (made from petroleum/oil), herbicides, and pesticides that we are exposed to. When our body is already inflamed from other irritants and our digestive tract allows toxins to enter our body, we have no way to know the damage they will cause. Many of these pesticides are neurotoxins, and can directly damage nerve tissue. They are a leading worry behind diseases like ADHD and Parkinson disease.

REDUCING INFLAMMATION

I hope you are now convinced that we need to generally be working to reduce inflammation in our bodies at all times because it causes so much cyclical damage. There are many things we can do to reduce inflammation in our bodies, and many of them go along well with our wellness practices.

Food

When using food to reduce inflammation the area, what we like to focus on is adding more antioxidants to what you are eating. Antioxidants fight off oxidants; so what are oxidants? Oxidants, also called reactive oxygen species (ROS), are the waste products that are made in your cells as a result of making energy, or adenosine triphosphate (ATP), to power your body. During normal function these build up in cells; they can cause mitochondria, the energy factory part of the cell, to be harmed. This can cause a person to feel fatigue due to lack of energy. Other symptoms include depression, digestive problems, headaches, muscle pain and weakness, and decreased mental function. Oxidant production is directly related to what you eat and the only way to reduce production is to reduce your caloric intake which is not always practical. Many inflammatory molecules, also act as oxidants and can be reduced through eating lots of antioxidant compounds.

Antioxidants are a category of substances that protect the pieces of the cells from the damaging effects of oxidants. Some of these substances include vitamin C, vitamin E, and selenium. They have this effect through what is called electron scavenging. When the oxidants are made they have an extra electron associated with them and this is what makes them damaging, that they could bond to anything. Antioxidants bind this extra electron to prevent it from reacting negatively within your body.

Good food sources of antioxidants include:
　　　Purple and red fruits and vegetables
　　　Orange and yellow vegetables
　　　Carrots, peppers, tomatoes
　　　Green tea
　　　Berries, beets, and grapes
　　　Apples, eggplant, grapes

TIP: Eat from the rainbow, if there is no color there aren't any good nutrients!

Papaya, broccoli, brussel sprouts, and strawberries are some of the foods highest in vitamin C. One papaya contains 300% of your daily requirement. One cup of strawberries contains about 140% of your daily requirements. Dark leafy greens and nuts are high in vitamin E. One cup of boiled spinach has almost 20% of your daily recommendations. 1/4c of almonds has almost 50% of your daily requirements. Seafood and other protein sources, including tofu, are some of the foods highest in selenium. 4oz of cod contains about 75% of your daily requirement of selenium. 4oz of tofu contains about 15% of your daily requirements of selenium. If you are in a constant state of inflammation, it would be an excellent idea to take more antioxidants than your daily requirement. The more the better.

Other than antioxidants, anything spicy will help increase your circulation and support moving blood, inflammatory cells, and healing molecules to where they need to go. Be sure to check the recipe pages in the back of this book to see some of our favorite dishes high in antioxidants and low in allergens.

What foods are you currently including in your diet that will reduce your inflammation?

What are your favorite antioxidant containing foods?

What are three meals you can make with high amounts of antioxidants? Try to eat one of these meals a day.

Choosing good fats over bad fats can also be a good way to reduce inflammation that is through your whole body. Most individuals end up eating foods containing high amounts of saturated fats. These are the fats that clog up our arteries, potentially damaging our heart They can even lead to heart attack and stroke if eaten in high enough amounts over time. There are much healthier options when it comes to what fats to eat.

Generally, you want to choose oils that are liquid at room temperature. When you think about fats in your body, they will not solidify in your arteries if they do not solidify on your counter. This then removes most of the fats that are used in all processed foods. Other than keeping it liquid, you want to lean towards vegetable oils that are high in omega-3 and omega-6 molecules. It is better to have a higher amount of omega-6 fatty acids and less omega-3s. Two good and popular oils for this are olive oil and coconut oil. Coconut oil is best to use for high heat cooking. I often substitute my oil in cooking with olive oil. Just note that usually I need a bit less oil in a recipe when I use olive oil.

When you choose these better-quality oils, your body will not only benefit from the good quality fats but it will also calm its inflammatory reaction. Inflammation is so common we get used to it always being there. This does not need to be the case.

Movement

When it comes to using movement to support reducing inflammation, it is quite easy. Get your body moving. This helps by increasing your circulation, and with chronic inflammation you need to keep getting oxygen and healing molecules to the injury and remove the inflammation. Inflammatory molecules will be 'disposed of' in the liver and kidneys to get them out of the body. The liver and kidneys 'clean' the blood and remove cells and molecules we do not want there. The kidneys concentrate these molecules into urine to be excreted and the liver uses them to create bile, which is helpful in digestion to break down fats. If urine or bile are not excreted properly, they too can cause damage and associated inflammation.

Movement also supports lymph drainage. Without movement this cannot occur effectively. Pathogens and other damaging molecules like to hide out in our lymphatic tissue and cause problems later down the line. By keeping your lymph tissue moving and getting toxins out of the body, movement can help reduce the potential for later problems. This is especially the case with the lymph tissue located under the arms in women. It is commonly discussed that increasing movement in this area can reduce the likeliness of problems associated with the breasts, where there generally is little movement of the associated lymph tissue.

Movement also increases our metabolism, breakdown and use of energy in our bodies. This is excellent to support our immune systems, because this added energy can be used to fight off infections when they first occur. Having consistent movement in your life will encourage a strong immune system in the first place, reducing the likelihood of going into a state of chronic inflammation. Movement also reduces our stress levels, reducing inflammation associated with the chemical byproducts of the stress system in our bodies.

Are you exercising enough to reduce your inflammation or do you still experience inflammation in response to exercise?

Hydration

Hydration generally supports the circulation and detoxification mechanisms of our bodies. Staying adequately hydrated will insure that when you increase your movement, your blood will easily be able to move, detoxifying both the liver and kidneys. Hydration, in conjunction with movement, can also support detoxifying our skin through sweating. Our sweat glands can hold onto toxin molecules if we do not sweat them out. Usually, they would just sweat away, but if you are not properly hydrated or haven't sweated in a while it can be important to do so. This is one benefit of using a sauna and why you should always shower afterwards. Sweating regularly can also generally improve the quality of your skin.

Sleep

Sleep is supportive of our immune system because when we sleep we are healing our bodies. That is what sleep is for. Your body needs rest to heal. This is the time that our bodies need to heal our acute inflammation challenges. When we hit a stage of chronic inflammation sleep will not be as directly effective. However, when you are in a state of chronic inflammation, sleep will continue to support reducing your stress level. This is an excellent area to manage inflammation in when it has become chronic, because added stressors will make inflammation worse and may be what is actually causing the chronic state of inflammation. Just get enough sleep and relax.

Are you getting enough water and sleep to support your wellness?

What wellness tools are you using now to lower your body's inflammation?

Are they supporting you? If not, what other tools could you use to reduce your body's inflammation?

CHAPTER 17: MOVEMENT PRACTICE STAGE 3

Homework Assignment 13

Follow weeks 1-3 of the movement practices as described in this chapter to learn more movements. Create a goal sheet and your own workout protocol. You can also choose to follow along with weeks 4-9 of the movement practices described here.

If you have been working on your movement since chapter 6 you are probably getting close to being ready for Stage 3 now. If you have already added in sun salutations on a regular basis you can now start to explore other methods of stretching and strengthening your body. If you are not yet at that point, do not worry. There will be time for you to come back to this chapter when you are. I do not recommend continuing with this chapter unless you are safely ready to do so. Feel free to now move onto the next chapter if you are not ready for this next stage of movement practice.

I have been doing regular cardio exercise at my moderate heart rate and I have previous experience stretching and strengthening.

There are two ways to incorporate additional and new general stretching and strengthening activities into your schedule. With option one you chose to, on an individual day, focus on a muscle group, doing both the strengthening and stretching exercises for that muscle group. Option two is to do a full body strengthening routine on day A and alternate with a full body stretching routine on day B. I personally prefer to do option one, that way if you need to skip a day for an unpredicted reason you do not suffer from balancing those muscles with stretching and strengthening. I have set up the following beginner stretching and strengthening patterns with this in mind. We will discuss repetitions of these exercises after.

Take some time as you read to practice each of these moves. There are many other movement options as well, but these will get you started without having to purchase any equipment or gym memberships. There are also many free online videos on how to do these activities.

LOWER BODY

Squats/lunges
Squats and lunges focus on the hips and quadriceps, the front and inner upper legs. The strengthening exercise is the squat.

To perform a squat, stand with your feet at a wide stance pointing forward with your feet parallel to each other. Raise your arms for balance and think first of relaxing your knees over your toes. Go slowly if you are not used to this movement. Think of your hips going down and backwards with your chest angling forward as counter balance. Do not bend more than your knees feel comfortable. Straighten your legs and relax your arms. You can do this and hold down, or do multiple repetitions. If you

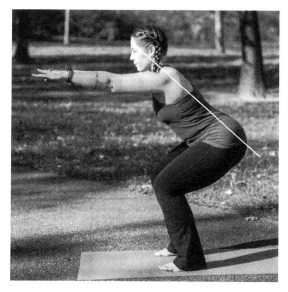

need to hold a wall or chair for support, be sure to have one available.

The same knee bending can be done with your feet pointing to the sides and your knees still going over your toes. It is best to do squats in both directions to work on the rotation of your hip joint. Most people are not used to this squat. Start with your feet at a comfortable outward rotation and remember to keep your knees over your feet. In the side squats you do not need to use your arms for balance. Think of your hips going straight down and not back, keeping your chest high and shoulders over your hips.

The stretching movement of these same muscle groups are our lunges. These too can be done forward, or to the side. With lunges, they can be done quickly as a strengthening exercise, but here we want to relax our muscles and hold the position until our muscles relax and stretch out. Begin with a forward lunge, keeping your hands on the ground at first with your front foot between your hands and your knee over your ankle (not your toes or further forward). Make sure your back leg is straight and your knee is off the floor if you can. You should feel a slight stretch in the front of your back leg, in your quadriceps muscles. If you do not feel a stretch with your hands on the floor and you can maintain balance, lift your hands to your knees, relaxing your shoulders and lengthening your back upwards. Hold until your muscle relaxes and the pain starts to go away. Don't worry, it will. If it is too intense, lower your knee towards the ground. Repeat on the other leg, taking a break between if necessary.

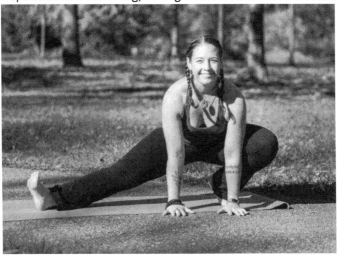

Side lunges can also be used as a strengthening exercise. There are two ways to do side lunges, and the main difference you will see is in the foot that is farther from the body. We will use the second kind in a little while. For this side lunge you are looking to stretch the outer side of the leg closest to your body, and the inner side of the leg farther from the body. Stand with your legs in a very wide stance, bend slightly forward for balance and bend one knee, leaning so your hip is directly over that foot. Hold this position until you feel comfortable there. Then shift your weight to the other side with your hip over your foot. If you do not feel a stretch with this alignment start with your feet further apart.

Leg lifts/Forward bends

We now move onto the back of the upper legs, our hamstrings. The stretch here is a very common one, however the strengthening exercise is not and it may take some time to get used to it. Do not worry if you struggle with this one, it is challenging to most people.

Let's get the strengthening exercise out of the way. To strengthen your hamstrings, it is easiest to lie flat on the floor, stomach down with your head resting on your hands. Trying to keep your bottom relaxed, lift one leg off straight of the ground. Hold it for a few counts and then lower the leg. Repeat with the other leg for one repetition.

If you find it difficult to lie flat on the ground, you can use a large ball, the edge of a low couch, a pile of pillows or similar to lift your body off of the ground. Make sure your back and hips are in a straight line. You do not need to raise your arms. Try to lift one leg at a time so that it is in line with the rest of your body. You may need to set up a mirror near you so you can tell if your leg is in line. We do not generally have this kind of special awareness of our bodies, so using a mirror for alignment here can be helpful.

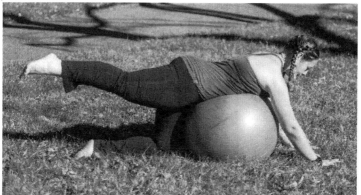

The most common stretch for the hamstrings and back of the legs is a forward bend. There are two ways to do this stretch, standing and sitting. With standing make sure your knees are slightly bent as to not put extra pressure on them. Allow your arms to relax and do not try to reach the ground, just allow gravity to pull your body downward. To keep your arms out of the way you can fold them over each other. Remember to relax your head as well. You can put blocks on the floor to put your hands on for extra stability if you need.

The sitting forward bend is recommended if you have any challenges with the standing forward bend. Try to keep your knees straight here and start sitting up straight and reaching your chest towards your feet. You can either relax your feet or use your muscles to pull your toes towards your face. This will offer an additional stretch if you are not as flexible yet. To receive the full benefit of this method, you will then need to relax your head down to your knees. If you are not yet able to have your body close to your legs, try the standing version of this stretch that uses more gravity to offer a stretch when flexibility is limited.

Leg lifts/heal drops

Most people, when they strengthen and stretch the lower body, they disregard the lower legs. These are two simple exercises that are done together to stretch and strengthen the front and back of the lower legs all at once. Stand with your toes on the edge of a stair, hold a railing for support. Practice doing these movements slowly with control for maximum benefit. Start by lowering your heels to relax your calf muscles on the back of your leg. Contract these muscles and slowly raise your heel as high as you can. With control, slowly lower your heels back down. Again, the slower you do this movement the more benefits you will receive.

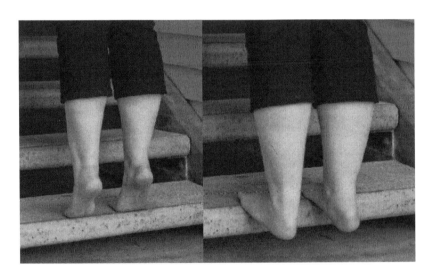

UPPER BODY

Neck lifts and stretches

With all of our computer usage, we tend to lose our neck posture and much of our stress is held in our shoulders as a result. There are two sets of exercises I recommend to start with (ignore the shoulders here for now).

Isometric contractions are contractions where you hold a body part still against a force trying to move it. To strengthen the neck, place the hand on the forehead, back of neck or side of the head. Push with your hand and use your neck muscles to stay stationary. Another option uses gravity to strengthen the neck muscles. Lying on your back or side, or on your hands and knees, move your head away from the ground to contract and lift the head. When bending the neck, do not think of bringing the head to the back or chin to the chest but rather straight ahead as in chin pointing towards the ceiling. Remember for both of these exercises to do equal repetitions to the front, back, and each side.

To stretch the neck while standing or sitting let your head relax and fold forward, to the side, or back. Relax the muscles and hold for the same number of seconds in each place. Take care when relaxing to the back and open the mouth to release tension on the front of the neck.

Push-ups/arm stretches

Most of us have done a push up before. There are a few key things to consider with your form to not injure yourself. Key things to look at include: keeping your hands under your shoulders, keeping your elbows close to your body, keeping your neck long and in line with your spine, and not dropping or raising your hips in relation to your spine and legs. If your arms are not strong enough to lower your body down, do not lower your body to your knees to do a push-up. This offers very little benefit. You will receive much greater benefits from holding a plank position with straight legs. When you need to rest from this position lower the knees and shake out your arms and try again with the number of repetitions you need. Remember in plank position to also keep your shoulders down. You can remind yourself of what this feels like by rolling your shoulders back when standing. This is a hard position of the shoulders to maintain and it is what offers the strengthening of the plank position.

To then stretch the arms you have a few positions and angles to choose from, most of which you are probably familiar with. Holding your hands with fingers laced, turn your palms away from you and push them away from your body out in front of you and then above you. This will stretch your shoulders together. A similar stretch with one arm at a time is to cross the arm across your body to your opposite shoulder. Using your other hand, pull that arm gently towards your shoulder. Repeat with the other arm. To offer a stretch to the outside and back of the arm, bend the arm above the head letting the hand drape behind the head. Using your other hand, gently pull from your elbow towards your free arm.

ABDOMEN

Front of the abdomen

When you did neck lifts, you keep the shoulders on the ground. Now is time to lift those shoulders off the ground for crunches. If your neck is not yet strong enough to lift your shoulders go the route of lifting your waist off the ground, rather than your shoulders, to strengthen your torso.

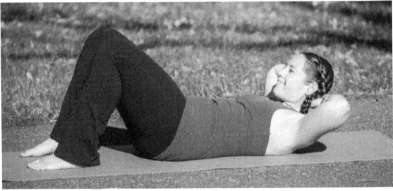

When doing a full crunch, I recommend having the hands at the ears, not holding the neck. Have your feet shoulder width apart. Think of bringing your chin up to the celling rather than bending your neck and bringing your chin to your chest. Lift your shoulders off the ground and think of bringing your chest to the ceiling. Relax down your shoulders down, relaxing your head and neck muscles between every contraction.

When your neck is not strong enough for this, you may try the method of doing a crunch by lifting your waist. Begin with your shoulders and neck relaxed on the ground. Lift your feet, bringing your knees to your chest. For some, the action of bringing your knees to the chest will engage your abdominal muscles in your stomach with this repetition. If you would like more of a challenge from this, bring your knees into the chest, lift your hips off of the ground, and lower your hips them slowly.

To then stretch out the front of your abdomen you will need to lie on your stomach and lift your shoulders off the ground with the help of your arms. Relax your elbows onto the floor and hold the position, relaxing the muscles around your stomach. If you need a deeper stretch you may push up your arms straight, locking your elbows. Remember for both of these to keep your neck long and in line with your spine. Do not strain your neck to look up and relax your shoulders down and away from your ears.

Back of the abdomen

After working on the front of the abdomen, stay on your stomach, to move into the strengthening exercises for the back. Think of this like a crunch for your back. Put your hands next to your ears again, relax your shoulders and legs, and keep your neck in line with your spine. You may want a friend to hold your feet down or stick your feet under a heavy object like a couch. Lift your shoulders off of the floor and, with control, lower back down. Breathe in before you lift. As you lift your shoulders, breathe out. This is very hard for most individuals because we rarely, if ever, do this kind of exercise in any class, program, or daily activity. This makes it even more important to do, because having a strong back from this strengthening exercise can help prevent throwing out your back later in life. It can also strengthen your back after an injury when done with proper supervision.

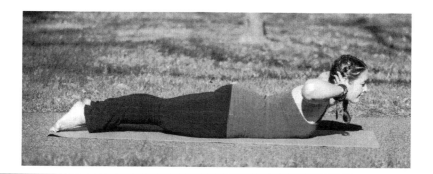

After you have done this strengthening exercise, follow with child's pose to stretch out the back. Sitting on your knees, extend your arms forward, stretching out the armpits as well, and relax the head down to the floor. Sit here for as long as you would like. This is the most comfortable relaxing stretch in this program.

Side bends

After you have done the front and back of your abdomen, you must also do the sides. These are some of the easy exercises because as you stretch between sides you are strengthening the opposite side. Standing, begin with your arms up at shoulder height with legs shoulder width apart. Move one arm upwards as you begin to bend away from that arm. Bring that arm close to your ear, trying to create a straight line from fingertips to your foot. Reach with the long side of your body in the direction of your stretched hand. Do not allow your body to drop to the side, instead keep your shoulders down and your body supported and stretching upwards. Keeping your arm and ear touching, lift your arm, head and body up to standing, again bringing both arms to shoulder height. Repeat stretching the other arm up to the other side. Return to center to complete a set.

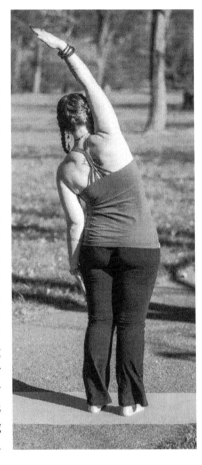

If you choose to do a slight alteration to this stretch, hold your arms together and stretch up with your feet together. This will give you a more intense stretch in your shoulders.

CARDIO

After you have increased your cardio to 30 minutes of moderate intensity exercise a day, continue with your cardio as you add in your stretching and strengthening exercises. This can add up to a total of 60 minutes of exercise a day into your life. It is great if you do an hour of exercise every day. You should also not let it stress you if you cannot get in a full hour every day. You have goals. Try to do as best as you can.

When you have reached thirty minutes of moderate intensity cardio exercise, and you are trying to save yourself some time with still getting recommended cardio exercise, you can increase to high intensity exercise some days of the week. Generally, the same benefits can be achieved from thirty minutes of moderate intensity activity as twenty minutes of high intensity activity. There are also other activities, other than walking, jogging and running, you can enjoy to achieve your appropriate time. Joining a community sports team is an excellent way to get your cardio exercise. Usually team sports also stretch and do some strengthening exercises before games so it is a great fun way to get all of your exercise for the day. Other great things include going to community social dances, taking exercise classes, water sports like canoeing, kayaking, and swimming, as well as hiking, skiing, and skating. There are so many possibilities.

What kind of exercises sounds fun to you?

What exercise would you like to do with other people? Who?

What steps have you made towards starting exercising at a higher level than you currently are?

REPETITIONS

When you are ready to work on the exercises in Stage 3, you will want to start slow. For the first 2-3 weeks follow the following recommendations for repetitions of each exercise. Make adjustments down whenever you need them. Make adjustments up only after the first week when you know how your body starts to heal in response to the exercise. Your body may not feel the results of the exercises until a day or two afterwards. This is why for your first few weeks you should keep a few days between working on the same body parts.

Weeks 1-3

Repeat days 1-3 with a day to rest in between for 3 weeks. (s=seconds)

	Exercise	Day 1	Day 2	Day 3
Lower Body	Forward Squats	3-5		
	Forward Lunges	20s each leg		
	Side Squats	3-4		
	Side Lunges	2-10s each		
	Back Leg Lift	3-4 each leg		
	Forward Bend	1 minute		
	Leg Lift/Heel Drops	2 rounds of 3		
Upper Body	Neck Press		2-5 second press	
	Neck Lift		3-5 each position	
	Neck Stretch		10s each position	
	Push-ups		3-5	
	Arm Stretches		10-15s hold each position	
Abdomen	Crunches			2 rounds of 8
	Abdomen Stretch			30s-1 min
	Back Lift			3-5
	Back Stretch			1 minute
	Side Bends			3-4 rounds

Be sure to take one day a week to rest from your stretching and strengthening activities, and continue your cardio exercises as you go. These stretching and strengthening exercises should not take more than 5-10 minutes each day. If you are able to keep track of how many repetitions you do on each activity, it is great to see your own progress over time.

This chart is to only get you started. Make changes as you need to target different areas of your body you feel could use more support. Do not add additional repetitions to do this. Add an additional set of the same number of repetitions. For instance, with the leg lifts and heel drops, you do three of each, twice. To target this area, do three sets, three times. When you can confidently do this you can move up to doing 4-2x to increase your endurance over this activity.

When doing repetitions of the same exercise take a rest between each set. This rest should be between 15-30 seconds to obtain maximum benefit from taking a rest between sets. Try not to wait longer between each set. Make sure to do the same number on each side of the body when it is called for, including both sides of the neck.

Weeks 4-6
Repeat days 1-3 with a day to rest in between for 3 weeks.

	Exercise	Day 1	Day 2	Day 3
Lower Body	Forward Squats	5-8		
	Forward Lunges	2-3, 20s each leg		
	Side Squats	4-6		
	Side Lunges	3-4, 10s each		
	Back Leg Lift	4-6 each leg		
	Forward Bend	1 minute		
	Leg Lift/Heel Drops	2 rounds of 5		
Upper Body	Neck Press		3-4, 5 second press	
	Neck Lift		5-8 each position	
	Neck Stretch		2-3, 10s each position	
	Push-ups		4-8	
	Arm Stretches		2, 10-15s hold each position	
Abdomen	Crunches			3-4 rounds of 8
	Abdomen Stretch			30s-1 min
	Back Lift			4-8
	Back Stretch			1 minute
	Side Bends			4-6 rounds

Weeks 7-9

Repeat days 1-3 with a day to rest in between for 3 weeks.

	Exercise	Day 1	Day 2	Day 3
Lower Body	Forward Squats	2 sets 5-8		
	Forward Lunges	3-4, 20s each		
	Side Squats	5-8		
	Side Lunges	3-4, 10s each		
	Back Leg Lift	5-8 each leg		
	Forward Bend	1 minute		
	Leg Lift/Heel Drops	3 rounds of 5		
Upper Body	Neck Press		3-4, 5 second press	
	Neck Lift		5-8 each position	
	Neck Stretch		2-3, 10s each position	
	Push-ups		2 sets 4-6	
	Arm Stretches		3, 10-15s hold each position	
Abdomen	Crunches			3-4 rounds of 12
	Abdomen Stretch			30s-1 min
	Back Lift			5-10
	Back Stretch			1 minute
	Side Bends			5-8 rounds

Continue to alter these as you need. By these 7-9 weeks you probably should be doing about 15-20 minutes of stretching and strengthening a day. With your cardio work outs, which you may be spending 20-30 minutes a day doing, you will be doing a little less than an hour of movement. These can easily be spaced through the day. Take your time.

WEIGHT LOSS

While most people think of dieting as the only way to lose weight, the only real way to lose weight or maintain a healthy weight is through a combination of healthy food choices and exercise. Conscious eating and movement practices guide you towards making choices that work best for your body. As you begin to include more exercise in your life, following this chapter and professional guidance, you may notice that your dietary needs may shift. Generally, if you will remember, to heal muscles after stretching and strengthening you will need to eat protein.

While you should be focusing your general food intake on fruits and vegetables, you may need to adjust the proteins you eat so your body can repair itself. Regarding cardio workouts, this is where your body needs its carbohydrates, the energy. These are your grains, fruits, and vegetables. You will want to ideally be eating these 60-30 minutes before exercise, and protein after exercise. Exercise can also help to relieve constipation. If you are looking for additional guidance to help you optimize your food intake with your exercise, please seek a dietitian and exercise professional to work with your specific needs.

HYDRATION AND SLEEP WITH EXERCISE

When you are exercising regularly, it is even more important to make sure you stay hydrated. There are calculations to figure out how much water you need to drink for the amount that you sweat, but it is much easier to just continue to drink while you are exercising. A good quantity judge is a cup every 30 minutes of exercise in addition to your normal water intake. Therefore, if you are normally drinking 8 cups of water a day you would want to drink 10 on a day you do an hour of exercise.

When it comes to sleep, you may find that you are falling asleep easier when you exercise. This can be a great tool to support your sleep patterns. Some individuals find that when they exercise right before bed they fall asleep much faster than they normally do. Experiment with what time of day is ideal for you to exercise, and use it as a tool to support your daily wellness.

CHAPTER 18: YOUR RELATIONSHIP WITH SPIRIT/DEITY/SOUL

Having already looked at your relationship with yourself and others, now an appropriate time to look at your relationship with spirit/deity/soul. When appropriate for your own needs, replace these words with ones that serve you. Each of us has the ability to experience something larger than ourselves and our community, but we all see that as a different experience. For some, there is a soul that connects everything in existence. For others, there are many spiritual beings greater then ourselves. This chapter is about your relationship with that which is larger than you. We all call it something different but here is an opportunity to see how your experience serves your greater being in the world.

LABELING

Just as we discussed with interacting with others, labels can mean a great deal to individuals. Take some time to look at how you label spirit/deity/divine/soul, and their relationship to each other.

What does divine/deity/spirit/soul mean to you?

Is there a place for divine in your life?

Does it serve you to label spirit with a name, face, history, or any other features?

Would it serve you to have a larger image of spirit?

EXPERIENCING SPIRIT

Is there a place for spirit in your personal environment?

How does this show up?

How does spirit show up in your daily life?

Do you communicate with spirit? How?

Does this serve you?

Where do you experience spirit? For some that may be a physical location, such as heaven or a beautiful park, for others they experience spirit in their cat or other beings and places.

How does spirit exist to you?

*Are there places where you **do not** experience spirit?*

RELATIONSHIP WITH DIVINE/SPIRIT

What kind of relationship do you look to have with divine?

*What do **you** do to support spirit/divine/deity?*

What does spirit/divine/deity do to support you?

What does worship mean to you?

> Worship: Reverent honor and homage paid to God or a sacred personage, or to any object regarded as sacred. To feel and adorn reverence or regard for. To attend service of divine worship.

Does this fit your definition and your interactions with divine?

How do you find joy in your relationship with spirit?

Just like we cannot have control over others we cannot, generally, have control over spirit. How do you respond when upset arises from something associated with divine or spirit?

PERFECTION

Can you accept that divine is not perfect?

What limits do you put on divine if you accept that it is perfect?

What new possibilities show up for you if you open to the possibility that divine is not perfect?

Would opening yourself up to this possibility serve you? Don't worry if it doesn't serve you. For many it won't.

RELIGION

What we have been discussing is our relationship to what we label as divine. Our world community has developed what we now call religion. While for some this is a set of their personal beliefs, for others religion is a structure of beliefs that has been developed by a community at large. These may or may not exactly fit your beliefs, and for some religions that is fine. For others, if you are part of that religion you must change your set of beliefs so that they are in complete alignment with the religious doctrine. Neither of these ways is the only way. To accept one another, we must accept that there is no one path but that we are all on our own paths through this world.

Do you participate in religion? If yes, how does this differ, if at all, from your interaction with divine?

Are there pieces of your worship that are missing from your religion?

Was your religion chosen for you or did you chose it based on your personal beliefs? How do you resonate with this idea?

GOALS

While some religions and individuals experience a spirit or deity this is not always the case. These following questions are to get you to think on how you interact with the divine.

What is the goal of the divine? Does it have one?

What are the goals of your interaction with the divine?

What do you want your spiritual practice to offer you?

What makes the divine important to you?

PARTICIPATION

Participation in a spiritual practice is almost always up to the individual. Every person resonates with a different level of connection to spirit, and this is the case in all personal and religious practices. This does not mean that the priest has a more important connection to spirit than a congregation (community united under common beliefs). They just have different levels of participation in their interactions with spirit. How do you interact with spirit?

How are you an active participant in your spiritual practice?

Does meditation or prayer have a place in your spiritual practice?

Would being a more or less active participant in your spiritual practice serve you?

In what other ways can you engage in spiritual practice?

SPIRITUAL WELLNESS

There are many common themes that show up in spiritual practices in relation to our other wellness techniques. Let's briefly explore these ideas and how they show up for us.

How do you experience food as spiritual nourishment?

How do you experience movement in relation to your spirituality?

Is there a connection between your spirituality and drinking liquids?

Is there a connection between your spirituality and meditation or breathing practices?

Regardless of your faith, spiritual beliefs, or path, we are all one. We all come from the same place, and are all going to the same place, even if we have different ideas on what those places may be. We all exists in the same realm. We are all made up of the same star stuff that existed many millennia before our life on our planet was even a possibility, and it will exist for much longer than we ever will. Things change, and we must accept that and be able to change with them. Just as religions and deities have come and gone over time, as our social experience evolves we must also evolve our belief systems to match.

Look to your own beliefs, needs, and relationship with others and spirit to help form how you interact with yourself, other individuals, and this world. It is through clear communication, open mindedness, and understanding that we will all make it through this world in a way we find successful. Please take some time to process some of the ideas in this chapter in relationship to how you view your relationship with yourself, your relationship with others, and your relationship with spirit. Are these relationships serving you and, if not, what can you do to improve these relationships?

CHAPTER 19: HERBS FOR WELLNESS SUPPORT

Many of the herbs listed here do not have dosage recommendations. This is intentional, as different products have different strengths. When using herbs, even for wellness support, consult with a practitioner on how much to take and what brands and sources are best for your specific challenges. When in doubt, ask. Many products will also have recommendations for use on the package. While not always the ideal recommendation, they are a good, safe place to start when determining how much of something you need to take.

SLEEP SUPPORT

In setting up your sleep schedule using herbs, there are a few things to remember from our sleep related chapters. Unless you are being consistent with both your bed time and your wakeup time, these products listed here will not be effective long term at creating a sustainable sleep schedule. There are many practices to include in your daily life to support a healthy sleep schedule before turning to using herbs. If you are actively practicing all of these, herbs will make those other practices more effective at developing a good schedule so you will be able to get the most out of your sleep.

After you have initiated all of the sleep support methods in this book, you may still struggle to set up a natural rhythm for your body to stick to. Using herbs and supplements can be beneficial at encouraging a rhythm in your body. Even herbs and nutritional supplements to support sleep should not be taken regularly. This is why setting up a consistent schedule is truly important to having your ideal night's sleep.

The herbs discussed here for sleep support should only be taken as long as needed and then promptly discontinued. While herbs are not generally addicting, we can start to rely on them and other natural supplements to get sleep every night, and over time this is an added cost you do not need to deal with.

Chamomile

There is no other substitution for an herb to help a child go to sleep. Chamomile is great for adults and children if you are just too awake and need help calming down. This is generally the challenge with children as they often are buckets of energy. For adults, when one cup of chamomile tea is not strong enough, you can take one cup an hour before bed and a second at bed time. A hops tea can also be effective for adults as it is a bit stronger. Hops is not necessary to use for young children.

Skullcap

Skullcap, used as a tea or tincture (alcoholic extract), before bed, helps to calm the mind. This herb is particularly supportive to take if you are having trouble sleeping because there are many thoughts going through your head while you are trying to sleep. This is not like a prescription drug and it takes some time for the body to accept that it is more relaxed and can take comfort in falling asleep.

Passionflower

Passionflower can really knock some people out, so take this in small doses to find what dose works best for you. This works directly on the nervous system to promote sleep. Use this herb if the others above are not supporting your sleep. This herb is one you do not want to take every night to help with sleep but only on individual nights when the others have not supported you in falling asleep.

Melatonin

Melatonin is not an herb. It is a molecule that occurs naturally in our body and rises in concentration in the evening as we go to sleep. It remains present in our bodies while we sleep, and helps us to maintain sleep through the night. When taking melatonin as a supplement there are a few things to consider. Melatonin supplementation can be addicting and with constant use your body can reduce its own innate production of melatonin. For this reason alone, as a natural supplement, it should be the last one you consider using regularly.

Melatonin comes in a variety of concentrations. The lowest ones of 0.5mg should be taken to support falling asleep. These are placed in the mouth and allowed to dissolve there for absorption through the tissue of the mouth for a more direct route to the blood stream. The higher concentration tablets are often enteric coated and should be swallowed. These will slowly break down through the night, and allow a constant supply of melatonin to support staying asleep through the night. Both of these methods can cause drowsiness the next day if not enough melatonin is used by the body at night. Please insure that you use these products safely, because even though they are a naturally occurring supplement, they are still drugs.

STRESS SUPPORT

Herbs can greatly support your venture to reduce stress in your life. While they are by no means a sole method of reducing stress they can support the associated physiological functions that are damaged by long term stress exposure. The general herbs we look at are called adaptogens and nervines. Some herbalists believe that some aphrodisiacs can also support stress management, but this is generally due to their relaxing effects which nervines also cover. The following adaptogens and nervines specifically support stress management.

While herbs can be great at supporting stress reduction, they are by no means the only way to improve your stress experience. Long term improvement can only be made through adjusting your entire life plan and interactions with the things causing you stress in the first place.

Ashwagandha and Ginseng

Roots of ashwagandha, Korean ginseng, and eleuthrococus (also known as Siberian ginseng) all can be protective against stress, particularly chronic stress. When these herbs are powdered, a teaspoon of one herb can be sprinkled on each meal for long term support. These are food herbs and do not have much of a flavor. Add at the end of cooking to not destroy the herbs with heat.

Ashwagandha is also an antioxidant and protects your nervous system from stress related damage. Ginseng specifically works on the cortisol system, the first stages of stress in our bodies. It also enhances memory, supports the immune system, improves blood sugar regulation, and protects the nervous system. Eleuthrococcus normalizes blood pressure and blood sugar. It can also support muscles as you add more exercise to your practice, improve memory, and support your immune system through its antioxidant actions.

Cordyceps

The mushroom cordyceps, powdered, can be added to soups with other herbal mushrooms to help tonify the nervous system from stress. It can also enhance sexual function and normalize blood pressure. Another mushroom, reishi, also protects the nervous system, supports the cardiovascular system, and generally reduces stress.

Green Tea

Green tea, drunk as a tea, is great for healing damaged tissues and protecting tissues with its antioxidant effects. It is anti-inflammatory, helps regulate blood pressure, and helps protect the nervous system. In general, green tea is thought to increase your life span. Keep in mind, green tea is high in tannins, and, if you remember for our earlier discussion, when you drink something high in tannins you should also drink an extra cup of water that day to reduce the effects of the tannins on your digestive system.

Holy Basil

Holy basil, *Ociumum sanctum*, is great at lowering stress-induced hormones and normalizing cortisol levels. It decreases the chance of getting gastric ulcers, normalizes blood pressure and blood sugar, it also generally elevates mood. My friends call holy basil, "a hug in a cup."

DIGESTION SUPPORT

Gentian

Gentian is an herb that is not talked about a lot because it is not used for much besides digestion support. Gentian is a classic bitter herb. Thinking back to when we talked about flavors, bitter stimulates digestive secretions, allowing you to break down your food more effectively.

Gentian does this very well in very small doses so no need to deal with the taste for too long. A few drops of tincture in your mouth 10 minutes before eating and you will be all set.

Ginger

This herb is a common one, and you probably don't usually eat it for its medicinal benefits, just for its taste. Like gentian it will stimulate your digestion, but it also calms an overactive digestive muscle as well. Ginger is commonly used for upset stomachs due to motion sickness. If you are noticing that you are having lots of stomach cramps and flatulence, you may want to add more ginger to your food. Keep in mind that these cramps may be a sign of a larger problem if adding ginger to your meal does not reduce their intensity.

Triphala

Triphala is actually a blend of 3 herbs from India. Together they balance your body's digestion very effectively. Most individuals who use triphala tables as instructed on the packages notice that their digestion becomes more regular. In other words, they start having regular and smooth bowel movements. If you are noticing that regardless of the food you are eating, you are still challenged by constipation, triphala may aid you in bringing your bowels back into sync.

Turmeric

This is another delicious culinary herb that you may not use frequently at supporting the digestive system. It is excellent at lowering inflammation of the intestines. If you are struggling with anything causing inflammation in your digestive tract, you may consider trying turmeric on your food. It goes great on just about everything from rice dishes, to eggs, and even on a popcorn snack. You can also use turmeric to support your stress response and nervous system.

Peppermint

While many people think of using ginger for stomach aches and motion sickness, peppermint does one better and supports these, as well as painful muscle spasms of the digestive system. If you feel that your digestion is more sluggish, you may want to stimulate it more with the ginger. If you notice instead that you need to cool down your digestion, peppermint tea is a good alternative to ginger.

Licorice and Marshmallow

While these are talked about in the next section on inflammation support, they also do a great job at coating and calming the digestive system as well. Remember, inflammation can affect all systems of our body and paying attention to where it is affecting us most can help us target what wellness practices will be most supportive to make a reduction inflammation.

INFLAMMATION SUPPORT

Most herbs and plant foods support a reduction in inflammation in our bodies. Some herbs do a particularly good job at it. These can be used on a regular basis by adding them to your food for daily support, or through taking a larger amount when you feel that you need additional support.

Garlic

One of my absolute favorite herbs is garlic. I know some people don't like the smell, but it really does wonders at fighting infections. As soon as I hear someone cough I start eating more garlic myself so I don't get sick. Garlic is great at getting deep in our bodies and killing things that are not supposed to be there. Garlic is antimicrobial and very stimulating to our circulatory systems. It helps kill those little buggers and then makes sure our body is clear of them. This makes it great for supporting inflammation and the immune system. It also is a pre-biotic, meaning it provides food to the good bacteria in our digestive tract. These bacteria help fight off the bad bacteria and create a calm environment that is less likely to become inflamed. So when our digestive tract is all inflamed, garlic can help feed the good bacteria and kill the bad bacteria, calming our inflammatory response in our digestive tract. To support your body with garlic in this way, eat one clove raw a day, unchewed, with honey.

Rosemary

Rosemary is another culinary herb that is great to use for inflammation. Not only does it directly support reducing inflammation, it is also a strong antioxidant herb. To get the antioxidant effects, add ½ tsp a day to your food, powdered. This will add a lot of flavor so be prepared. You can also get its anti-inflammatory effects by drinking a rosemary tea made from 1-2 tsp of rosemary leaves. Having this daily will support your overall inflammatory state.

Calendula

Calendula, another favorite herb of mine, is great at full body inflammation. Calendula is a flower that is best made into a tea with a small handful of flowers a day (5-10 grams or about 1/4-1/2 cup of dried flowers). Their beautiful orange colored flower helps support the liver to detoxify our blood. Calendula is also thought to support the quality of our skin because of its detoxification effect. It also calms our inflammatory system by reducing the production of inflammatory cytokines, the ones that signal for more inflammation to occur. This makes it great for use in chronic inflammation because it lowers the molecules that make the inflammation reoccurring. Calendula also is great at improving the strength and quality of our blood vessels, supporting circulation.

Chamomile

For children who experience mild inflammation, chamomile can be a great calming anti-inflammatory herb. Chamomile tea, with a few teaspoons of flowers, is great for children and can also be used for stomach aches. Skullcap, a plant in the mint family, also has mild anti-inflammatory actions. It is also calming, like chamomile, and they could be used together for a regular tea to take daily to keep yourself, and your immune system, calm.

Licorice and Marshmallow

Licorice and marshmallow are two good anti-inflammatory root herbs. Take 1-2 tsp and boil the roots in water for 15 minutes to make a decoction to strain and drink. While licorice is a sweet herb it can raise blood pressure so take care with this. Marshmallow, while not sweet, is very sticky and not everyone likes its texture. It is called a mucilage herb and helps to calm inflammation in the digestive tract simply by creating an environment to calm the local inflammatory response.

While all of these herbs can be used to lower your inflammation, they should not be used without professional supervision and all of the other wellness techniques described through this guidebook. Continue to explore how your body works, what it feels like, and how it is affected by the different things you do. Our bodies are constantly changing, and we will need to keep changing how we interact with our own bodies and others as a result. Explore, have fun, be happy, keep moving and above all stay well.

APPENDIX A:

THE NEXT STEP ON THE WELLNESS PATH

If you are looking to continue on your wellness path, there are many options you can take. Here are some resources you can follow, separated out over a variety of the wellness practices we discussed in this book. When not listed, all of the referenced organizations and centers can easily be found by searching online by profession and professional organizations, as their web addresses are likely to change over time.

NUTRITION COUNSELING

If you are looking to further your work on nutrition it is not difficult to find a nutritionist. The Certified Board of Nutrition Specialists is an organization present in at least sixteen states that certifies nutrition and wellness practitioners. These are not necessarily dietitians. Dietitians focus more on medical conditions and supporting them with supplementation, often in a hospital setting. While a dietitian may serve your needs, if you are looking for support similar to what you have found in this book you would likely prefer working with a nutritionist.

If you are unsure about the quality, ability, and validity of the practitioner you are choosing to work with, be sure to ask about their credentials and explore for yourself if they will work for you. Keep in mind that unless the individual is also certified or holding a degree in the subject, a nutritionist or dietitian should not be recommending movement or herbs to you.

PERSONAL TRAINING

It can be really hard to exercise with a strange person you do not know. Working with a personal trainer, however, should be one of the easiest steps to take after completing this book. Personal trainers are very helpful at supporting your movement path and finding ways to help you overcome your challenges in a safe and effective manner. They will be essential in supporting weight loss or additional strengthening you need beyond what this book has to offer. Personal trainers are able to look at your current abilities and design work out movements that are doable for you, and will directly send you towards your personal goals you have determined throughout this book.

Personal trainers can be found at just about any gym. Some gyms may not hire professional, certified personal trainers. Be sure to ask about the credentials your personal trainer has and make sure that they are current, not expired. One of the top certifying boards is the American College of Sports Medicine, or ACSM. Compared to many personal training programs, the ACSM requires thorough physiology and safety training for all of their trainers, and is the reason I recommend you look for a certified personal trainer associated with ACSM.

Unfortunately, you may have noticed during one of the movement practice chapters that you are not ready for adding more movement in your life due to health challenges. If this is the case, you should consider getting a recommendation from your doctor on a personal trainer who is also certified as an Exercise is Medicine professional. These individuals are trained to work with slightly more at-risk populations. They can target support for different health challenges in which movement may potentially be detrimental. The ACSM has three different levels to their EIM certification. Finding which skill level EIM professional you need to work with can be discussed in a private session with one of these individuals.

Keep in mind that a personal trainer, unless also certified or holding a degree in nutrition, should not be recommending food therapies to you.

WELLNESS COUNSELING

There are a large number of individuals out there that call themselves wellness practitioners. This is usually a nonsense term and does not mean the same to two different people. While this entire book has been centered around wellness, there are very few educational programs that prepare an individual to become solely a wellness counselor. This does not mean that there are not individuals that are well qualified to support you in your journey. Each wellness practitioner is going to have a certain focus so look for one that specializes in an area you need additional support in. If you have completed this book you are much further along in your path than you realize.

The ACSM is currently in the development stage of having a certification for wellness coaches, however, as of the fall of 2016 it is not yet in existence. Be sure to clarify the skills of the practitioner you are planning on working with, and know how they can clearly support you before starting on that path. Also keep in mind that wellness counselors are sometimes also called life planners, and may just focus on organizational and stress reduction skills which may be exactly what you are looking for.

SPIRITUAL, PSYCHOLOGICAL, AND STRESS SUPPORT

Even I feel uncomfortable with the idea of going to a psychologist but sometimes it is necessary to get your stress and mental well-being under control. Most pastoral programs also include a small amount of psychological support training, so if you are a spiritual person this may be an avenue that works for you. Additional stress management programs exist and should be considered when you are also working with a psychologist.

Participating in a week or weekend retreat can do wonders for our own psychological well-being. One center I recommend exploring is the Omega Center in central New York State. While it may be a trek for you, they offer a large number of retreats that may serve your spiritual, psychological, and stress related challenges. If their location does not work for you, they are able to put you in touch with similar centers in your region.

HERBAL MEDICINE

If you are interested in looking more closely at how herbal medicine can support your wellness you have a small number of options. The American Herbalist Guild is the governing body of herbal medicine in the United States. When looking to work with an herbalist for wellness and herbal support, look for an individual that is a Registered Herbalist, RH, with AHG. There are less than 500 in the United States, and you can find them through the American Herbalist Guild website.

There are a number of individuals in the United States that label themselves as 'Master Herbalists.' Unfortunately, this is a term that does not have much backing to it, and just about anyone can pay for an online course and call themselves this without any real training. There are now two graduate degree programs in the United States where individuals can obtain a Master of Science Degree in Herbal Medicine. If you are looking for a more medicalized version of herbal medicine, as presented in this book, look for an RH with AHG or for an individual with an MS in Herbal Medicine or Herbal Therapeutics as it is more recently being called.

There are many herbalists that are less scientifically minded. This is not to say that their practices should be ignored. Herbal medicine has a long-standing tradition in our world, and most things individuals will tell you about herbs have some grain of truth to them. A number of herbalists work more with the spirit of the plant, some with the energy of the plant, and homeopaths work with even more minute plant and nutrient vibrations to stimulate changes in the body. While each path is different and may work differently for you, take some time and shop around before finding an herbalist that is right for you if you are looking for more than the chemical actions of herbs in your body.

If you are looking to work with some of the herbs recommended in this book for wellness support these can be purchase at a number of quality places online. Some of my favorite brands for purchasing teas and tinctures include Mountain Rose Herbs, Herb Pharm, Oregon's Wild Harvest, and Starwest Botanicals. Some of these can be purchased in local health food stores, but generally you can purchase larger quantities for less online.

If you have any other questions regarding herbal medicine, please do not hesitate to be in contact with The Dancing Herbalist. We can be reached through our website **www.thedancingherbalist.com** and through **info@thedancingherbalist.com**. We offer a number of free herbal classes on our website as well as a plethora of information we post regularly on our blog.

APPENDIX B:

ADDITIONAL NUTRITION EXPERIMENTS

FOOD EXPERIMENTS

The following pages include a variety of food experiments for you to try to help you target if you need to make any alterations in your normal food patterns. Continue to keep a journal so you can determine any additions or subtractions from your normal regime that would serve you.

The goal of this is to continue to help you observe what you are eating and how it can change how you feel. Use these experiments as opportunities to experience foods in a different manner. Explore how you feel by answering these questions: How are you feeling both physically and mentally? Are you happy, sad, mad, somewhere in between? The more detailed you are the more you will be able to learn from the experience. I suggest trying at least one or two of these experiments so that you are able have some practices to start. It is completely appropriate to try each of the suggested foods in each experiment over time for more learning.

1. Protein

Choose one protein source below. Have this be your primary source of protein (from the list) for two days. Answer the questions below:

> Red meat (including hamburger, steak, ham)
> White meat (including chicken, turkey)
> Vegetarian Protein (tofu, beans, nuts or other)

What protein source did you choose and why?

How many times a day did you eat this?

How did your body feel before you ate the protein?

How did your body feel after you ate the protein?

Was there a change?

How did you feel when you went to bed in the evening?

How did you feel when you woke up in the morning?

Would you continue to eat it after this experience?

2. Fruits

For two days, eat three pieces/servings (think 1 handful) of fruit a day, six total servings of fruit. Some fruits are suggested here. Try different kinds of fruits. Answer the questions below.

> Apple, pear, peach, strawberries, blueberries, raspberries, black berries, pineapple, cranberries, raisins, grapes, apricots (All can be fresh or dried but fresh is preferred in general. When the only option, frozen is preferred to canned.)

What fruits did you choose?

What made you choose these fruits?

What did you enjoy about your experience with these fruits?

What did you not enjoy about these fruits?

How did your body feel eating this much fruit?

What would you do differently with eating fruit in the future?

3. Breakfast

For three days in a row eat a good breakfast that includes at least two of the following types of food: protein, fruit, vegetable, grain. Below are some suggestions:

> Toast with peanut butter, waffle with strawberries, apple with peanut butter, vegetable omelet, beans and rice, granola with cranberries.

What do you normally eat for breakfast?

What did you choose to eat for breakfast?

How did you feel after each meal?

How did you feel three hours after each meal?

What was your favorite breakfast you ate and why?

Was there anything about eating breakfast that was not positive for you?

Did you observe any difference in your experience with different kinds of foods?

Would you continue eating this breakfast? Why or why not?

4. Five meals a day

For two days, eat five meals a day. A meal can be anything from an apple with peanut butter, veggie sticks with hummus, to a hamburger with French fries, or Lasagna with salad. Just eat a total of five times in one day.

List your 5 meals for each day (record as you eat them):

What was your favorite meal and why?

How did your body feel when you went to bed on day 1?

How did your body feel when you woke up on day 2?

Was there a difference on the night of day 2 or the morning after? If so what was it?

Did your body react differently to any one meal?

Would you continue to eat this frequently? Why or why not?

5. Try a new vegetable

As odd as it sounds, try something new that you don't remember having had before, or something that you previously did not enjoy. People's tastes change over time and most people enjoy having a variety of food in their diet so trying new things is essential. This can be cooked or fresh.

What new vegetable did you choose to eat? Why?

How was it prepared?

Would you continue to eat this vegetable?

Would you prepare it any other way or eat it with other foods? If yes, how and which ones?

Are there other vegetables you would like to try? What are they?

What do you like or dislike about vegetables?

How could you use this to incorporate more new vegetables into your diet?

Have you observed any new food interactions you were unfamiliar with from these practices?

Other options

There are many other options of experiments you can do around your food choices. As soon as you begin to regularly explore how your body feels, you will be more in control of your own choices and be able to effect both your mood and physiology through your food. Make up your own experiments based on what you have already observed and always record your findings so you can see your progress and track patterns. You can also consider trying one of the following food related experiments.

1. Have breakfast every day.

2. Exercise before eating.

3. Have a glass of water before and after each meal.

4. Stop eating 3 hours before bed.

5. Remove a food from your diet.

If you are choosing to remove a food from your diet, it is highly recommended that you do this with the direct help of a nutritionist or another qualified practitioner. You want to be sure that you are still getting all of the required nutrients from your other foods.

When removing a food, it will take a length of time for your body to get back to its normal state if the food has been causing a problem. You may not notice all of the changes, and this is to be expected. Plan to not eat that food for at least a month to know for sure if it is causing a problem for you. When you choose to re-introduce the food into your diet, be sure to do it in an environment where there are others that can support you. It is not uncommon to have a very serious reaction when you re-introduce a food you have a sensitivity to.

APPENDIX C:

RECIPES

Choosing to change your eating habits is one of the hardest things to do when you can no longer eat a food that you had frequently. To get you started, here are a few of my favorite allergen free recipes. Many of these recipes do not have exact ingredients. This is purposeful to get you to explore how to cook, and experience your food in a way that works for you.

I have not included any dishes containing meat. Let's be honest, most of us are good at eating enough meat. I have only included two of my favorite main dishes here for you. For most individuals, while having a vegetarian diet may be helpful it is not necessary for long term health. There are a number of easy meat dishes that can be prepared in a healthy fashion and combined with the side dishes here for a full meal. Remember, one of the best food choices you can make is to focus eating vegetarian-like dishes and supplementing them with meat as needed.

So, let's get cooking!

SNACKS

Cheesy Kale Chips (vegan, gluten free, dairy free)

Ingredients

- 1-2 bunches of kale
- 1c cashews (pieces are fine)
- 2-3 cloves of garlic
- 1/2c lemon juice
- Olive oil
- Salt

In a blender, combine the cashews, garlic, lemon juice, a few dashes of salt (as desired), and enough olive oil to get the mixture to blend smoothly.

Have ready a baking sheet with parchment paper ready, and preheat your oven to 250°F. In a large mixing bowl, rip up your kale into chip sizes pieces, removing the middle vein. Discard the vein or use in compost. With about ½ of your kale in the bowl, scoop ½ of the cashew batter onto the kale. Using your hands, massage the batter on all sides of the kale, mixing well. Lay the kale out on your parchment paper being careful not to overlap chips too much. Overlapping or clumps of batter can cause the chips to be partially wet and they may mold after a day or two.

Put in oven for 45-60 minutes, until all chips are crisp. Remove from oven, allow to cool and store in an airtight container on the shelf. If not all of your chips dry completely, these chips can be kept in the fridge. Dried chips may get soggy in the refrigerator.

Hummus (vegan, gluten free, dairy free)

This hummus makes an excellent vegetable dip, addition to salads or Mediterranean cuisine, as a substitute for mayo on sandwiches, or an excellent protein to put in vegetarian sandwiches.

Ingredients
- 1-2c chick peas (dry or canned)
- 2-3 cloves of garlic
- Olive oil
- Salt
- Water*

Optional Ingredients
- Roasted red peppers
- Sun dried tomatoes
- Basil or Pesto
- Jalapenos or other peppers

If you are using dry chick peas (or any other beans), start by soaking your beans for at least 24 hours. Cover them in water and drain, and rinse, recover every 6-8 hours. After you have done this, thoroughly rinse the dry beans and put them in a pot with water. Simmer for 1-2 hours over medium heat until cooked. About 1 cup dry chick peas will yield 2 cups cooked. Drain and allow to cool completely before blending. To save you time, after you have cooked the beans you can choose to freeze portions of them for later batches of hummus.

Add your cooked or canned chick peas (drained) and your garlic to a blender. Add salt as desired and start with a splash of olive oil. Add water to make creamier, and more oil as desired to build more richness to your hummus. When you have reached your desired texture in the blender, add any of your optional ingredients to taste. You may choose to add more salt at this stage as well.

*Note: The more water you add the faster this hummus will go bad. It is recommended to use your cooking water or water from the chick pea can for this.

Herbal Popcorn (vegan, gluten free, dairy free)

Popcorn is not hard to make itself, but there are endless options on how you can dress it up. If you have an air popper, I highly recommend adding olive oil or butter to your popcorn after popping so that these delicious herbs stick more effectively to the popcorn.

To pop popcorn on the stove top:

Use a large stock pot with a tight lid. Start with putting 6 tablespoons of olive oil or coconut oil into the pot with one kernel of popcorn. With the lid off, turn on medium heat and wait for that one kernel to pop. This will tell you that the oil is hot enough to add the remainder of your popcorn.

Quickly pour in your popcorn so that a full layer of kernels covers the bottom of the pot. Cover and continuously shake the pot over your burner. It may take a minute for the kernels to start popping, but keep shaking the pot so that the kernels do not stick to the bottom. They will eventually start to pop. Keep shaking on the heat until you only hear kernels popping every 3-5 seconds. Remove from the heat and quickly pour into a large bowl. I have noticed that even 5 more seconds in the pot can cause popcorn to start to burn and stick to the pot. With this method, you will not need to add more oil to your popcorn for the herbs to stick.

Herbs!!!!

I recommend using powdered herbs on popcorn but you do not need to do this. Dried onion and garlic pieces work great too. Here are a few of my favorite combinations. You can find a handout at **www.thedancingherbalist.com** for even more popcorn ideas.

Immune Support Popcorn

Sprinkle on your popcorn dried turmeric, garlic, and onion powder. I like to add some Celtic sea salt to this as well for the added minerals. This blend is great, and works as an anti-inflammatory popcorn for snacking at exercise heavy events.

Digestive Support Popcorn

Add powdered rosemary, basil, and a lot of ground black pepper to your popcorn. You can also choose to use lemon zest or lemon juice sprinkled over the popcorn.

Dessert Popcorn

Combine on your popcorn: powdered peppermint, cinnamon, and cocoa powder. You may also choose to add a dash of dried maple sugar or a drizzle of honey if you don't mind it being a bit sticky.

BREAKFAST

Vegetable Pancakes (vegetarian, gluten free option, dairy free option)

Ingredients (single serving)

- 1 egg
- Splash of milk (almond milk or kefir work well too)
- 2 tablespoons flour (chick pea works well)
- Vegetables
    - Carrot
    - Onion
    - Summer Squash
    - Potato
- Soy sauce
- Maple syrup

Thinly slice or julienne your vegetables and lightly sauté them with a splash of olive oil. For one pancake you only need about 5 slices of each vegetable or they won't be covered in batter. While those cook, mix together your one egg, flour, and enough milk to thoroughly moisten. I recommend mixing with a whisk to more easily break up flour clumps.

Spread vegetables out on sauté pan and pour batter over the top to make one large pancake. Cook on medium heat. This batter will not rise and will form more of a crepe like pancake. In a small dish, mix soy sauce with a splash of maple syrup for a dip. When you see small holes forming in the top of your pancake batter, you know it is time to flip it over. You may choose to put some more olive oil around the edge of pancake to prevent it from sticking on its second side but this is not necessary.

Remove from heat, slide pancake onto a plate and serve with the maple soy sauce on the side. This recipe is easily made larger for more individuals. I cooked this for a whole camp site once and it was a huge hit with my friends. The chick pea flour with almond milk and egg made a great high protein breakfast that was a bit different than the normal fare.

MAIN DISHES

Butternut Squash Soup (vegan option, gluten free, dairy free)

Ingredients

- 1 large or 2 small butternut squash
- 1 large onion
- 2 large carrots
- 2 medium potatoes
- 2 full stalks of celery (about 10in long)
- 4-8 cups chicken or vegetable broth*
- Salt

Peel, de-seed, and cube your butternut squash. Put in large stock pot with about 2-3 cups of your broth. Start to steam them. Add in your other vegetables, chopped and NOT peeled. When not peeling vegetables, be sure to wash them thoroughly. When you cut your celery, cut it in about ¼ inch to ½ inch wide pieces. You will be glad you did; your soup will be less stringy. If you like a thicker soup you can consider adding another potato. With all of your vegetables in the stock pot, cook until all are tender, adding more broth as needed.

When your vegetables are cooked, let them cool slightly and have a separate large bowl ready. When you can handle the pot easily, put your vegetables into the blender in batches, removing them when blended to the separate bowl. When all vegetables are blended, stir soup together so all pieces are incorporated, adding salt to taste.

I usually eat it at this point and think the creaminess is perfect. You can choose to melt some butter into your soup or pour in a bit of cream, but these are not necessary for the deliciousness of this soup.

*I highly recommend using chicken broth if you are not vegetarian because it really adds a depth to the flavors of the soup.

Zucchini Pie (vegetarian, gluten free option)

Ingredients

- 1 super large zucchini or 2 medium size zucchini (about 3 cups grated, yellow squash also works)
- 1 large onion
- 1 cup of homemade pesto*
- 1 cup flour (can be gluten free)
- 3 eggs
- 1 cup mozzarella or provolone cheese shredded
- 1 teaspoon baking soda
- Salt and pepper to taste

Make your pesto, grate your zucchini or squash, chop your onion, and mix it all in a bowl. Put it all into a large pie plate and put it in the oven at 350°F for 45-60 minutes. It is done when golden brown on top and a toothpick comes out clean. I recommend letting it cool for 15-20 minutes before cutting. It can be served warm or cool.

This is my absolute favorite summer time dish with fresh pesto. I have friends that will drive an hour to come get a plate of this, even when it is not fresh from the oven. Nothing compares to this vegetable filled, cheesy, eggy, basil goodness.

*I highly recommend making fresh pesto for this. It can be expensive to purchase basil to do so. Personally, I grow basil each year just for making this dish. You can find a recipe for my pesto by visiting my blog at **www.thedancingherbalist.wordpress.com** and searching pesto.

SIDE DISHES

Coleslaw (vegan option, gluten free, diary free)

Ingredients

- ½ medium or 1 small cabbage, green or red
- 3 carrots
- 1 large onion
- Mayo (or vegan mayo)
- White vinegar (or other vinegar)
- Sugar
- Dried mustard
- Paprika

This is the one salad I make with a homemade dressing at home. I never understood, growing up, why my grandmother called mayonnaise a salad dressing. This coleslaw does just that.

Cut your vegetables as small or as large as you like. My mother makes her coleslaw by running her vegetables through a vegetable grinder. I prefer to have nice large chunks of cabbage. Mix your vegetables together in a bowl.

In a separate bowl, add a dollop of mayo with equal parts white vinegar and sugar, just a splash. You do not need much of this dressing. It should be a thin dressing. Add dried mustard and paprika to taste. Pour over your vegetables and mix. Your vegetables should be lightly coated and much of your dressing should fall to the bottom of the bowl.

I think this coleslaw is best on day two in the fridge. Just mix up the bowl again to re-dress the vegetables and enjoy the flavorful crunch of the veg with the sweet tangy dressing.

Roasted Root Vegetables (vegan, gluten free, dairy free)

Ingredients

- Vegetables of your choice
  - Onion
  - Potato
  - Beets
  - Winter squash (acorn/butternut)
  - Carrots
  - Parsnips
  - Rutabagas
- Olive oil
- Seasonings of your choice
  - Garlic
  - Rosemary
  - Parsley
  - Sage
  - Thyme
  - Lemon zest or juice
  - Pepper
  - Salt
  - Maple syrup

This is a super simple recipe that has lots of options for you. When you are practicing conscious eating techniques, learning to combine recipe ingredients together to form your own combination is an excellent cooking practice.

Preheat your oven to 350°F and prepare a baking sheet with a layer of aluminum foil. Peel and chops your vegetables of choice into bite size chunks. Toss in a bowl or on your baking sheet with some olive oil. Spread out your vegetables and allow to roast for about 40 minutes or until all vegetables are tender. Be sure to check the tenderness of each type of vegetables as they may cook at different rates.

When your vegetables are cooked, remove the pan from the oven and put all of the vegetables into a bowl. Toss on your seasonings, and don't be shy about it. One good way to decide on what seasonings to use is to smell them first. If they smell good to you there may be some nutrients in there that your brain is saying you need. Always remember to also add salt and pepper, to taste, at the end or you may allow your family or guests to do this as they choose.

Some of my favorite combinations include:

- Beets, onions, lemon, and thyme
- Potato, onion, garlic, rosemary, and sage
- Carrots, squash, parsnips, garlic, thyme, and a drizzle of maple syrup

Sweet Chard Sauté (vegan, gluten free, dairy free)

Ingredients

- 1 bunch of swiss chard
- 1 medium onion
- Olive oil
- Sunflower seeds
- Dried cranberries
- Salt and pepper
- Your favorite spice blend.

Cut up your onion and get it sautéing in your pan with some olive oil. Cut your chard, including the stem, perpendicular to the stem, into ½ inch strips. When your onions are starting to become translucent add your chard to cook. It will slightly wilt.

When your chard is cooked, throw in a handful of sunflower seeds and a handful of cranberries long enough to warm them up. Add salt and pepper to taste and add some of your favorite spice blend. I like to use an onion and herb mixture I have to top off this dish.

I really enjoy serving this dish to people who do not eat greens often. Compared to many leafy green vegetables, chard is not quite as scary for some reason. This recipe is also sweet and crunchy with the cranberries and sunflower seeds, making it fun for kids to get their daily dose of green vegetables.

Zucchini Casserole (vegetarian, gluten free)

This dish was one that I grew up having every summer with my parents. It is delicious both hot and cold, and there are a few different ways you can make it. See what you like best to share with your whole family. The cheese makes this one delicious for kids.

Ingredients

- 1 medium zucchini
- 1 large onion
- 2 medium tomatoes or 1 can juiced tomatoes
- 1/2 cup to 1 cup shredded mozzarella or cheddar cheese
- Olive oil
- Salt and pepper

Begin by slicing your zucchini into rounds and your onion into strips. Sauté these on medium heat with some olive oil. If you are using fresh tomatoes, cut them open and remove the seeds. Run the seeds through a mesh strainer to retain some of the juices. Discard the seeds.

When your zucchini and onions are transparent, add your tomatoes. Cook long enough to allow the vegetables to absorb some of the liquid remaining. Sprinkle cheese over the top and allow to melt and mix in. This will also absorb some of the liquid. Add salt and pepper to taste and serve.

DESSERTS

Apple Crisp (vegan option, gluten free option, dairy free option)

Ingredients

- 6-8 apples
- 1 stick of butter (dairy free works well)
- 1 cup flour (gluten free works fine)
- 1/2 – 3/4 cup sugar
- Powdered cinnamon

Peel and slice apples. Pile them into a small baking dish. Pour a splash of water over the apples. Thoroughly sprinkle cinnamon over all of the apples. Many recipes call for only 1 teaspoon of cinnamon. I tend to use closer to 1-2 tablespoons. Cinnamon really helps your body to process the high sugar content in the crust.

In a separate bowl, cream together the butter, flour, and sugar. You can choose to add more or less sugar here as you desire. More sugar will make for a crunchier crust. Crumble this mixture over the top of your apples. I find that if I use dairy free butter it is more of a solid rather than a crumble crust, but that is just fine.

Put in an oven at 350°F for about 45 minutes, or until the edges of the baking dish start to bubble slightly. Allow to cool slightly before serving. If you can handle more sweetness you can top this with a scoop of ice cream or homemade whip cream, but this is by no means necessary.

Flourless Chocolate Cake (vegetarian, gluten free, diary free option)

This recipe was one I came across in my e-mail one day years ago. It comes from the Gluten Free & More magazine. They have an excellent free subscription to their recipes, and if you are experimenting with different food choices I recommend seeing what recipes they can offer.

Ingredients

- 1 cup whole almonds
- 3/4 cup unsalted butter (can be dairy free)
- 1 cup sugar
- 4 large eggs
- Vanilla extract
- 1/2 cup cocoa powder
- Raspberry puree (optional)
- Salt

Heat your oven to 325°F, and toast all of your almonds for about 10 minutes. In a grinder, grind 2/3 of your almonds. Separately, chop the remaining and keep them to the side.

With a fork or pastry cutter, cream your butter and sugar together. Mix in ground almonds. Add one egg at a time, a splash of vanilla, salt, and finally your cocoa. Lightly grease a small baking dish. I use a loaf pan. Pour in batter and sprinkle remaining almonds on top. Bake for about 40 minutes or until a toothpick comes out clean.

While you allow it to cool you can make a raspberry puree to use as a sauce. Simply blend a few fresh or frozen raspberries with a few tablespoons of confectioners' sugar and a splash of lemon juice. Slice the cake and serve with a drizzle of raspberry.

Roasted Cinnamon Pears (vegan, gluten free, dairy free, sugar free)

Ingredients

- Pears (1 pear makes two servings)
- Cinnamon
- Canning rings
- Dark chocolate bar (optional)

You can probably come up with this one on your own, but it is still delicious. Slice a pear in half; remove the core with a melon baller or spoon. On a baking sheet, place canning rings upside down and place your pear in this ring, cut side up. Sprinkle on some cinnamon and pop in the oven. When you notice that the pear is becoming juicy you can remove them from the oven and enjoy like so.

You can also go a step further and place a square or two of your favorite dark chocolate in the hole you cut after the 10-15 minutes in the oven. Return the pears to the oven and allow the chocolate to melt. When melted, be very careful removing them from the oven. The rings will help to prevent the pears from tipping and spilling the lovely chocolate everywhere. This decedent desert can also be sprinkled with espresso powder instead of cinnamon if desired.

APPENDIX D:

HOMEWORK ASSIGNMENT OVERVIEW

Through this book there are a number of suggested assignments for you to work on. A separate workbook is available to guide you in these assignments and can be downloaded or purchased at www.thedancingherbalist.com. Do not feel like you need to move quickly through these assignments as they are a life of practice in themselves. Commit to practices as they feel appropriate for you as you move through this book.

Assignment 1

Observe and record the following for a week.

- When you drink water
- How much water you drink?
- When you urinate
- The color of your urine on a 1-5 scale

Do you notice any patterns?

Did you notice any other symptoms through the week that could be associated with your hydration level?

Assignment 2

Observe and record the following for a week.

- What food you eat?
- How much of each food?
- What time you eat?
- Anything else that goes in your mouth: all drinks, cigarettes, gum and mints, medicines, and supplements.

Assignment 3

Choose one of the hydration techniques from this chapter and choose to follow it for a week. Record in your journal what worked well for you and what challenged you with the hydration technique. Numbers 1, 2, 3, and 4 are recommended.

Assignment 4

Do you have a water bottle yet? Keep it filled all week and no more than 10 feet from you at all times. Having it available makes all the difference.

Track how many minutes of movement you do every day until you hit 30 minutes for 5 days in a row. This is any kind of movement and can include things like standing and doing dishes.

Assignment 5

Observe and record the following for a week as you practice breathing and meditation for sleep support.

- When do you start getting ready for bed?
- When did you get into bed?
- What time did you fall asleep?
- What time did you wake up?
- What time did you get out of bed?
- How many times did you wake up during the night that you remember?
- How long you were awake when you were up in the middle of the night?

Assignment 6

For a week you will spend time preparing for bed. To make sure we do this practice well we will give ourselves two hours before bed with no work and no screens, television, computer, phones, or otherwise. Take this time to read, meditate, take a bath, shower, enjoy a dessert or beverage, prepare clothes and supplies for the next day. Start to turn the lights off around your home so you can enjoy the dim light of the evening. Take two hours to relax. Continue to record the same journal. This may be really hard to find the time to do for most of us, especially if you have kids and they require attention too. You can make this a family time, but make sure it is important and know it is relaxation time, not running around time. This is an experiment to observe how your body experiences sleep with extra 'me time' prior to sleep.

Assignment 7

Observe and record the following for a week.

- What food did you eat?
- How much of each food?
- What time did you eat?
- How do you feel physically after each time you eat food?
- How do you feel emotionally after each time you eat food?

Practice using the physical and emotional feeling words separately for your experience of your food. After each day, record any patterns you notice with how you 'feel' in relation to food.

Assignment 8

For two weeks, do a full set of sun salutations twice, minimally, a day. They can be at the same time. Record how your muscles feel before and after this practice each day.

Assignment 9

For two weeks, set an alarm to wake up at the same time each morning, even on days you have off. Record what time you go to bed and how you feel in the morning.

Assignment 10

Go back and review all of your food related journal entries. Look through them and see if any patterns emerge of foods that are supporting you and ones that are not supporting you. Choose one food to eat more of and one to not eat at all. Continue with this choice for 2 weeks and record how you feel after meals in response to your change in meal plan.

This assignment may be one that you need to repeat over and over again until you find that you are having pleasant experiences after all meals.

Assignment 11

Observe and record the following for a week.

- What caused you stress today?
- What actually happened? What was the phenomena?
- What choices could you make so this would not stress you?
- What choices could you make to remove this challenge?
- Would these changes serve you?

Assignment 12

Choose one flavored water at the end of this chapter and choose to make this. Substitute one non-water drink you have a day with this flavored water or tea for one week. In your journal, record how easy or hard it was for you to make this change. Would you continue to substitute your beverages for water? What would make it easier for you to do this?

Assignment 13

Follow weeks 1-3 of the movement practices as described in this chapter to learn more movements. Create a goal sheet and your own workout protocol. You can also follow along with weeks 4-9 of the movement practices described here.

APPENDIX E:

GLOSSARY

A

Acidic – An environment with more hydrogen, H⁺ molecules; has a pH of 0-6. Examples of acids are citrus, vinegar; some parts of the human body are more acidic, like the stomach, so that it can digest food and nutrients.

Acute - A sudden condition, as opposed to a long-term condition. Breaking a bone is an acute condition; a long-term one would be if the bone healed improperly, causing permanent problems.

Adaptogen - Any natural herbal substance that helps the body adapt to stress.

Adhesive - A sticky substance.

Anesthesia gas - A gas that places the individual into unconsciousness so that they do not feel pain. Used before surgery.

Angiogenesis – Growth of new blood vessels.

Antioxidant - Molecules that destroy oxidants. Found in a lot of fruits, and some oils (i.e. olive oil). They have a positive effect on the body.

Atom – A small particle in chemistry. For example, a water molecule has three different atoms, two hydrogen and one oxygen, which each have electrons, protons, and neutrons.

B

Basal pulse rate – The lowest heart rate you experience. Normally found when first waking up in the morning before moving.

Bicep – A muscle with two large pieces. If you look at your arm, between your elbow and your shoulder, the muscle closer to your body is a bicep.

Brain wave - Electrical signals in the brain. A machine can be used to detect the different kinds of brain waves in your brain while you are awake, asleep, under the effect of certain drugs, etc.

C

Cardio - Exercise that raises the heart rate.

Cardiopulmonary system - Lungs and the cardiovascular system together.

Cardiovascular system - Consists of the heart, veins, and arteries of the human body.

Chronic - A long-term condition; may sometimes be permanent. Diabetes, osteoporosis, and other conditions for which there are no "cures" are considered chronic.

Cohesion - Forces between molecules that hold together liquids and solids. Water has this property, which is why there are not just water droplets floating everywhere; it binds together to create bodies of water.

Consciousness - The state of being aware rather than not paying attention.

Contemplation - The act of considering something; takes more attention and concentration than everyday thinking.

Contraction - When a muscle shortens, usually to bend a joint.

Cortisol - Otherwise known as the stress hormone; the hormone produced by the adrenal glands when one is anxious or stressed.

Counter balance - When the weight of one thing balances the weight of another. If you are wearing a purse on one shoulder, a counter balance to the weight would be a purse on the other shoulder at the same time.

Cytokine - Molecules that help regulate the actions of the immune system. They are indicators of an immune response.

D

Deionized - Removal of ions from a substance.

Desensitized – A decrease in sensitive to a particular action/substance. This occurs after repeated stimulation by a substance, causing the body to no longer be effected by it.

Detoxification - Process of removing toxins from the body. This can be done through sweating, bowel movements, and urination.

Detoxification systems - The systems in the human body that rids the body of toxins. These systems include the hepatic system (liver), urinary system, digestive system, the skin, and lymphatic system.

DI water - Deionized water; water that has either been processed to remove all bacteria, minerals, and all molecules that are not H_2O, water. Normal water contains a variety of minerals. DI water acts like dry water and will seek out nutrients to add to it. This is distinct from filtered water; filtered water filters out sediment, visible items, and some chemicals, but bacteria and minerals can still exist. Filtered water should typically be safe to drink, bathe, and cook with; DI water is used for making medicines, certain health practices like neti pots and breathing machines. It is not safe to drink.

Diarrhea - When bowel movements are very loose or watery. This can be caused by certain foods, allergies, or illness.

Digestive system – The organs of the human body that are involved in the digestion of food.

Diuretic – A substance that increases the amount or frequency of urination. Caffeine, from coffee or tea, is considered a diuretic.

E

Electrolyte - A nutrient required by the body to stimulate energy production within all cells of the body.

Elimination - The act of getting rid of waste products, generally, as a bowel movement.

Enteric coated - When a pill has an external layer that prevents it from being broken down by gastric acid.

Enzyme - A molecule that helps a chemical reaction to take place.

Evaporation - When a liquid, usually water, turns from liquid to gas. For example, the steam that rises off of water when it boils.

F

Free weight - Weights not attached to a machine that can be moved by the body for exercise.

Fibrous tissue - Tissue that is made out of bundles of a substance called collagen; typically, very tough and durable. Tendons and ligaments are made of this as well as the filler tissue between our organs and muscles.

G

Gene transcription - The first step in gene copying. A piece of DNA is copied into messenger RNA. The mRNA takes the copied segment to another part of the cell to be build a protein from the RNA code.

H

Hamstrings – A group of three muscles that are located on the back of the thigh. They allow you to lift your leg behind you.

Hibernation - When a metabolism temporarily slows down, generally with lower temperatures.

High intensity heart rate - Heart rate that is at 85% of your maximum heart rate. When exercising, this is generally the amount of exercise when you can neither sing or talk.

Hydrogen - The lightest chemical element known by the chemical symbol H^+

Hydrogen bond - A bond between two hydrogen atoms that are not in the same molecule. This is a gentle bond that easily breaks and reforms. It is due to hydrogen bonds that water molecules line up against each other and form a cube like structure when frozen.

Hydrophilic - A water loving substance; easily absorbs and mixes with water. Hydrophilic is the same thing as lipophobic.

Hydrophobic - A water-repelling substance; unable to mix with water. An easy example is oil. Hydrophobic is the same thing as lipophilic.

Hydroxide – The molecule OH- (oxygen and hydrogen together) with a slight negative charge. Hydroxide molecules will easily bind with free hydrogen that is positively charged to balance its charge.

I

Immune system - The system of the human body that fights diseases and infections.

J

Joint capsule - Packaging that surrounds specific joints like the knee. The capsule provides nourishment and protection for the joint to allow it to move more freely and effectively. The capsule can become damaged and inflamed, causing pain.

Julienne - A way of cutting vegetables: cutting them into long, thin strips.

K

Kinetic energy - Energy an object has when it is in motion. Ex: the energy a ball has as it rolls down a hill due to gravity.

L

Leukocyte - A white blood cell; cells in immune system that are "first responders" to infections/diseases.

Ligament - A band of collagen fibers that connects bones to other bones.

Lipophilic - Lipid loving substance; substances that dissolve in lipids, also known as fats or oil like substances. Lipophilic is the same thing as hydrophobic.

Lipophobic – A lipid repelling substance that will not mix with fats or oils. On example is water. Lipophobic is the same thing as hydrophilic.

Low intensity heart rate - Heart rate during low intensity activity, like sitting or standing in place, generally under 45% of our maximum heart rate.

Lymphatic system – A system in mammals that collects waste molecules in lymph nodes. This waste is ';/transported through lymph vessels to be deposited back into the blood stream for filtration by the kidneys and removal from the body.

M

Maximum heart rate – The highest heart rate your body can handle without passing out. This is determined either by mathematical estimation or through a stress test for a more precise measurement.

Meditation - The act of relaxing your mind and body so that you can observe your thoughts.

Membrane - A flexible tissue that separates two environments. For example, your skin is a membrane between your other layers of skin and the outside world. Membranes allow some materials to pass through while preventing others.

Metabolism – The act of digesting molecules to produce energy. This is done both in our digestive system and individually within each cell to produce the energy each cell needs to live.

Microbiota – The collective term for microorganisms in the human body. For example, the gut flora, or gut bacteria that helps break down food. Not all microorganisms are health positive and therefore supporting the growth of good flora is helpful for maintaining wellness.

Moderate heart rate - Heart rate during exercise generally identified as 65% of your maximum heart rate. This is observed by the ability to talk while exercising but not being able to sing.

Mucous membranes - A layer tissue that secretes mucous to lubricate and moisten the area tissues. The most commonly known mucous membranes are in the mouth, nose, and female genitals. The digestive tract also contains mucous membranes to help food pass more easily through the intestines.

Musculoskeletal system - The entire system of bones and their respective muscles in the human body.

N

Nervine - (noun) A drug/substance that acts upon the nervous system. (adjective) Medicinally acts upon the nerves; tends to refer to quieting nervousness, anxiety, and stress.

Neuron - A cell in the nervous system that transmits a signal to or from the brain.

O

Osmotic balance – When the balance of dissolved molecules is equal in concentration on two different sides of a membrane.

Oxidant- A molecule byproduct of a chemical reaction in the body. Oxidants can sometimes cause damage in the body and it is recommended to eat foods high in anti-oxidants to neutralize the effects of oxidants.

Oxygen - Chemical element. Combined with two hydrogen atoms, it makes a water molecule.

P

pH scale - A scale from 0-14 that measures the acidity/basic of water (or other substances). A substance is more acidic if it has more H^+ molecules, and basic if it has more OH- molecules. Anything from 0-6 is acidic, 8-14 is basic, and 7 is neutral. Water has a pH of 7.

Physiology - Branch of biology; the connection between the observed physical actions and underlying chemical changes. One easy example would be dehydration, when the lack of water cause physical changes to the body.

Pilates - A technique invented by Joseph Pilates that focuses on using the body weight to stretch and strengthen all muscle groups in the body.

Pillars of wellness – The separate actions that contribute to our wellness. These are different for each of us but generally include hydration, nutrition, sleep, movement, social interactions, and stress reduction.

Plank - Physical exercise in which one holds a pushup position for a long period of time. If your wrists are weak, you can do this position on the forearms instead.

Polar - A molecule that has one positive side and one negative side. They commonly line up, attracting a negative and positive end, respectively.

Q

Quadricep - A muscle that has four large pieces. The muscle group on the front of your thigh is a quadricep, or your quads, and when contracted, allow you to lift your leg to the front.

R

Respiratory system - The system of the human body concerned with breathing. Primarily concerns the lungs and the muscles needed to breathe.

Reverse osmosis - When a solution is forced through a semipermeable membrane that does not allow minerals and bacteria to pass through. This is a method used for such processes as filtering water.

S

Shavasana - Also known as the dead man's pose; a yoga posed typically used at the end of yoga practice to help bring on meditation. This position is lying on the back with feet at shoulder width and relaxed to the sides. Arms are relaxed about 6 inches from the body with elbows straight and palms upwards.

Solvent - A liquid in which molecules dissolve.

Stimuli - Anything that has influence/impact on a particular system. For example, a baby's cry may stimulate the nervous system and make an individual immediately run to see what is wrong.

Stool - Feces or excrement produced from the digestive system. Most people call it poop.

Strengthening - Any activity that makes the body part more able to withstand force. This is done through repeated contractions of a muscle. The healing process promotes the muscle to be stronger.

Stretching - Elongating a muscle. Pulling it to release tension. Should be done gently before and after exercise.

Stress response - Otherwise known as the fight or flight response; happens when a human encounters a situation they find threatening/harming.

T

Tannin - A molecule that gives the dark color to coffee and tea. It is used to tan leather and can have similar action on the digestive tract in high enough quantities. It has a dry taste.

Tendon - A tough band of *nonflexible* collagen based tissue that connects a muscle to its associated bone.

Toxin - A substance that either is or can be detrimental in a biological system, like the human body.

Triceps - A muscle with three large pieces. If you look at your arm between your elbow and shoulder, the muscle that is more towards the back of your arm that connects, over your shoulder blade, to the back of your neck, is called the triceps.

U

Universal solvent - Solvent that dissolves more than any other liquid. Water is the universal solvent.

Urogenital system - Organs in the urinary and genital system.

V

W

Wellness- The quality or state of being healthy in body and mind, especially due to the result of deliberate effort. An approach to healthcare that emphasizes preventing illness and prolonging life, as opposed to treating diseases.

X

Xylem - Tissues in plants that are responsible for distributing water and minerals from the roots the rest of the plant.

Y

Z

JILLIAN CARNRICK first became interested in plants in high school, where she took her first botany class. Jillian attended Maine Central Institute, an international boarding school in central Maine. There, she was not only introduced to many international students, but also became deeply involved in the school's ballet academy and environmental science program. Being inspired by these three communities, she earned a Bachelor's Degree in Biology with minors in Asian Traditions and Dance at Muhlenberg College. Completing a capstone project on Chinese Medicine, she was introduced to the East West School of Herbology. Under the guidance of Michael and Leslie Tierra she began her studies of herbs. After college, she moved to attend classes at the Maryland University of Integrative Health. There she studied under herbalists such as Bevin Claire, Camille Freedman, Kevin Spelman, James Snow, James Duke, and Simon Mills and graduated with a Master's of Science in Herbal Medicine in 2012.

During graduate school, Jillian continued her studies of dance and became a Certified Personal Trainer with the American College of Sports Medicine. Upon graduating from MUIH, Jillian opened The Dancing Herbalist, LLC. This topical products company combined Jillian's passion for dance and movement, her skills as a Certified Personal Trainer, and her love of crafting high quality products. With this company, Jillian is continually researching the best herbal extraction methods as well as new modes of herbal absorption through the skin. Her desire to find the best traditional herbal formulas, combined with her knowledge of scientific developments, has led to many successful products including her Ylang-Ylang Rose Geranium Cream, winning an award at the 2012 American Herbalist Guild Symposium.

Jillian has been continuing her research on various traditional uses of herbs, and now works to relate this information to modern clinical research being done on these herbs. Most recently, Jillian presented two posters at the American Herbalist Guild Symposium in 2014. Jillian's poster, "Arnica: Friend or Foe", received the award for "Most Clinically Relevant." This poster broke down the traditional uses of non-homeopathic arnica, and looked at the modern research on how this plant extract works in the body. Jillian also searched for the safety indications that traditional herbalists were using. She was able to relate these indications to modern clinical trials to determine a safe and effective way of using arnica both internally and externally. She now continues to research herbs used topically to find new and interesting ways of making topical products for healing support. Her learning has continued from there, obtaining a level 1 Exercise is Medicine credential through the American College of Medicine in the spring of 2016. Ever learning and loving life, Jillian is glad every day to get to share her knowledge with all communities she walks into, supporting the wellness of those around her.

Feel free to follow Jillian on the following social media platforms:
Facebook: The Dancing Herbalist, LLC (business page)
The Dancing Herbalist's Herbies (group)
Word Press: The Dancing Herbalist
Twitter: @DanceHerbalist

Jillian publishes a free monthly wellness newsletter listing her classes and upcoming events. You can sign up for this by visiting her website at www.thedancingherbalist.com.

Made in the USA
Middletown, DE
27 December 2016